STRONG
MEDICINE

STRONG MEDICINE

The Ethical Rationing of Health Care

PAUL T. MENZEL

New York   Oxford
OXFORD UNIVERSITY PRESS
1990

Oxford University Press

Oxford New York Toronto
Delhi Bombay Calcutta Madras Karachi
Petaling Jaya Singapore Hong Kong Tokyo
Nairobi Dar es Salaam Cape Town
Melbourne Auckland

and associated companies in
Berlin Ibadan

Published by Oxford University Press, Inc.,
200 Madison Avenue, New York, New York 10016

Oxford is a registered trademark of Oxford University Press

Library of Congress Cataloging-in-Publication Data
Menzel, Paul T., 1942–
    Strong medicine : the ethical rationing of health care /
Paul T. Menzel.
        p. cm.
    Bibliography: p.
    Includes index.
    ISBN 0–19–505710–4
    1. Health planning—United States—Moral and ethical aspects.
2. Medical economics—Moral and ethical aspects. I. Title.
    [DNLM: 1. Cost Control. 2. Ethics, Medical. 3. Health Policy—
economics—United States. 4. Health Services—economics—
United States. W 50 M551s]
RA395.A3M46 1990
174′.2—dc20
DNLM/DLC
for Library of Congress   89–16007 CIP

9 8 7 6 5 4 3 2 1

Printed in the United States of America
on acid-free paper

for Susan

Preface

Early in 1988, the Oregon legislature affirmed an administrative decision that the state's Medicaid program[1] should no longer cover heart, liver, bone marrow, and pancreas transplants. Averaging more than $150,000 per procedure for a projected thirty recipients a year, these expensive remedies were deemed unaffordable, at least compared to the prenatal care for more than 1,500 women that could be funded in place of the transplants.

One of the people waiting for a liver transplant who consequently never got one was a thirty-six-year-old single mother. Her fourteen-year-old son attended the Oregon hearings. He heard the lofty ideals cited in favor of the prenatal program and the denials that anyone here was "playing God"—they were only doing what had to be done for the public good. To the son, however, the senators must have seemed like God.

Interestingly, the president of the state senate who led the fight against providing the expensive high-tech procedures was a practicing physician. "If we pay for transplants now," he said, "we will put a very small Bandaid on a very large iceberg" of people without care. His opponents called him "Doctor Death." One bitterly rejected his "abstract discussion" about saving more lives another way. The state administrator who initially proposed cutting transplant funding, though, was hardly abstract or insensitive. On her desk she kept a picture of an adorable seven-year-old boy, one of the potential recipients who died after the legislature's decision.[2]

This is only one of many possible cases in which rationing health care presents moral difficulties. The essential sort of dilemma raised by all rationing cases is classic: how do we treat with dignity and genuine respect the individual who gets tragically shortchanged by a policy that seems best overall? If it is economic efficiency that leads us to choose that policy, then the conflict lies between the demands of efficiency and commitment to the individual patient. Both sides of that conflict pull hard on our moral sensitivities, so we may just want to compromise between them. Yet we want a true reconciliation, not an unstable cease-fire or some question-begging "victory" for either side.

Such a fundamental reconciliation, I will argue, is possible—not always but certainly sometimes. Cost containment does not have to be just a cliché mouthed by budget-constrained administrators, heartless legislators, or narrow-minded economists. Under the proper conditions it can represent respect for the hard trade-off preferences of patients as persons. If individual patients beforehand would have consented to certain policies of denying marginal procedures, those policies would appeal to far more than some economist's or manager's fascination with aggregate "efficiency." They would appeal to respect for patients as persons who make these hard choices themselves.

How far can this line of thought carry us in decisions about scarce resources in medicine? It is largely this question that has led me to write this book of connected essays. Sometimes my conclusions endorse economic efficiency; at other times they do not. An implicit theme throughout is that we should neither blindly follow nor blindly reject considerations of economic efficiency. To avoid those two narrow channels we very much need an ethical framework for making rationing decisions. If we use our heads and think hard about what rules we really want to govern our lives, I argue that we will selectively restrict what we do to promote and preserve life and health. That, of course, will be strong medicine to swallow, but, backed up by individuals' consent, there is nothing morally crude, cheap, or callous about it.

Chapter 1 examines several ways of looking at the health-care provider's basic moral conflict between commitment to individual patients and the socially efficient use of resources. Individuals' prior consent to less than maximum health security for their futures, I argue, allows the best resolution of this conflict. Chapter 2 attends to the philosophically fundamental issue beneath that argument: whether it is morally legitimate to cite persons' presumed consent to risk to justify policies that later happen to work to their disadvantage. Chapter 3 focuses on the particular problem of putting a monetary price on life, and then Chapter 4 takes up a fascinating question about how to compute the cost of saving lives. If we extend smokers' lives, for example, by persuading them to quit, do we have to include as a cost of our action their later "normal" expenses from living longer, such as pension support and health-care expenditures? Chapter 5 critically applies prior consent reflections to an existing model for measuring quality of life and making more efficient rationing decisions—"quality-adjusted life years." Chapter 6 focuses on one of the most disconcerting and difficult contexts for rationing policy: imperiled newborns. And Chapter 7 proposes a way of thinking about what would be an equitably efficient level of care for the poor. Chapter 8 takes up several nasty problems exacerbated by competitive forces in the current American health economy, and Chapter 9 defends a conceptual strategy for responding to the serious threat to effective cost containment posed by malpractice suits. Chapter 10 draws together consent considerations with other ethical distinctions to argue for expanding our supply of transplantable organs with a procedure usually thought to dilute the role of consent: "routinely" taking people's cadaver organs unless they object beforehand. Finally, Chapter 11 defends a qualified version of the threatening notion of a duty to die cheaply.

Throughout I presume that we confront a situation of scarce economical resources for health care. Some will charge that such a presumption already reflects mistaken social priorities. Daniel Callahan rightly rejects "guns versus canes" objection to health-care rationing which he sums up as follows: "if we can afford to spend more than $300 billion on national defense each year, another $25 billion on tobacco products, and $500,000 for one Super Bowl commercial, why should we entertain . . . any serious discussion" of cutting back on expenditures for beneficial medical care?[3]

Like Callahan, I would reject this objection. His reasons are entirely adequate. (1) "The fact that worse economic villains can be found" does not justify burying our heads in the sand about how we use our valuable health-care resources. (2) "One of the prices of democracy is that people are allowed to have other needs and interests than those of health and health-care delivery," no matter how much we may disagree with the way they get prioritized. (3) The tolerance of taxpayers is limited, so while a reduction in medical expenditures admittedly does not guarantee that the savings will be spent wisely, "an escalation of spending . . . almost ensures that money will not be adequately available for other needs, including those of children."[4]

Rationing exists already in the actions of insurance companies, legislatures, hospitals, physicians, and individual premium payers. The demands of efficiency are here to stay, from market competition to government regulation. We need to get on with the public business of determining how we should handle all of this ethically.

Tacoma, Wash.   P.T.M.
March 1989

NOTES

1. In the United States, health care for welfare recipients.
2. Specter (1988). The quotations of the state senate president, John Kitzhaber, are from Specter's article. See Kitzhaber (1988) for his own developed views on the larger issue.
3. Callahan (1987), p. 126. Callahan's context is specifically the restriction of expenditures on the elderly; mine is broader.
4. Callahan (1987), pp. 127–28.

Acknowledgments

In writing, just as in medicine, resources used may exceed value produced. From one point of view, the present volume might be a case in point: a year's time and sabbatical salary, one major grant and several small ones, two summers, countless evenings, and so on. But from another perspective, the process itself made the whole project worthwhile. The research and writing took me first to a charming English university and then to an idyllic writer's hideaway, the ideas that proliferated were invigorating, and the collegial support I enjoyed throughout was rich and assuring.

The whole project would have been impossible without a full year's sabbatical support from Pacific Lutheran University and the National Endowment for the Humanities (grant FB-24867-87). Several chapters were shaped by a semester's residence at the University of York's Centre for Health Economics; its director, Alan Maynard, provided a gracious welcome. While I was there, John Bone, Roy Carr-Hill, Anthony Culyer, Christine Godfrey, Melanie Powell, and Alan Williams kindly commented on early chapter drafts. Faculty advancement awards from Pacific Lutheran University, the American Lutheran Church, and the Burlington Northern Foundation made the extended visit possible.

For various aspects of special assistance, I thank Charles Bergman, Dennis M. Martin, Carolyn Schultz, Robert Veatch, Albert Weale, and Daniel Wikler. Some superb critics helped out on particular chapters: George Agich, Stanley Brue, William Knebes, Ronald Moore, Haavi Morreim, James Muyskens, Gunnulf Myrbo, David A. Peters, and Norris Peterson. At Oxford University Press, editor Jeffrey House contributed valuable suggestions, and Wendy Warren Keebler transformed a clumsy and idiosyncratic manuscript.

At my home university, Kay Whitcomb and Opal Huston assisted in the initial preparation of the manuscript and bibliography. And throughout, Susan, Tam, Heidi, David, and Matt all too often put up with disrupted mealtimes and rude silences as I found myself lost in QALYs, the costs of smoking, or whatever.

Two of the chapters have been adapted from prior publication: Chapter 3 from "Prior Consent and Valuing Life," in George Agich and Charles Begley, eds., *The Price of Health* (Dordrecht: D. Reidel, 1986), pp. 91–111; and Chapter 8 from "Economic Competition in Health Care: A Moral Assessment," *Journal of Medicine and Philosophy* 12 (February 1987): 63–84.

Contents

STRONG
MEDICINE

1

Could an Economist Take
the Hippocratic Oath?

The Conflict

In the best of all possible worlds both economic efficiency and commitment to the individual patient would govern the delivery of medical care. In the real world the conflict between these two factors is increasingly disrupting the health professions.

On the one hand, the traditional primary allegiance of health-care providers is to their individual patients: they cannot deny patients something they think would genuinely help. The doctor's Hippocratic oath illustrates this.[1] On the other hand, we all endorse the sensible goal of economic efficiency, getting the greatest value from our resources. We want to get the most health for our health-care dollars and to obtain as much value from every extra bit we invest in medicine as we could get by using the required resources on something else entirely. In economists' jargon, we want to minimize our opportunity costs.

This conflict is sharpened considerably by the financial context of modern medicine. Once a patient is insured, the patient's interest typically lies in receiving the best possible medical care regardless of whether the resources thus used might produce greater benefit elsewhere. The moral and professional allegiance of clinicians then seems to collide head-on with wider economic efficiency. Efficiency will sooner or later call for restricting care that would benefit individual patients. This is "hard efficiency": it is surely not just the elimination of waste, and it leaves the health economist at seemingly irreconcilable odds with clinicians and their oath.

When each side in such a stark conflict has so much intuitive appeal, it is

hardly surprising that the ensuing debate is heated. The traditional conception of loyalty to the individual patient even if that leads to sacrificing some
of the overall value of resources gets ardently defended even by those who
call for identifying and curtailing unnecessary procedures. Wasteful practices
must be eliminated, says Marcia Angell, but "the physician cannot serve two
masters—his patient and society's coffers. . . . We [in the medical profession]
should . . . argue for spending whatever is necessary for effective medical care.
Our responsibility as individuals is to each patient."[2]

Most economists, on the other hand, feel that physicians must stop treatments "when marginal benefits equal marginal costs."[3] The medical profession's mistaken conception of clinical freedom has usurped "democratic
power in the name of doing good for the individual patient. . . . The individual patient has inevitably been willing to play along since it is in his interests
(selfishly) to do so."[4] British economist Alan Williams argues the point
trenchantly: if practitioners "regard . . . cost as 'not germane to ethical medical practice,'" then what they really believe is that when one person stands
to benefit, by no matter how little, "there is no limit to the sacrifices that
others may properly be called upon to bear." That is not "ethics," Williams
notes; it is "fanatics." Morality itself demands hard efficiency.[5]

The problem will not go away in the natural course of events. Commitment
to patients is not likely to diminish. If anything, the continued solidification
of the informed consent requirement is moving us toward an increasingly
patient-centered ethic. Commitment to the patient is also surrounded and
nourished by a wealth of themes and images deeply embedded in medical
culture. Not the least of these is the military metaphor for medicine: "Disease
is the *enemy,* which threatens to *invade* the body and overwhelm its *defenses.*
Medicine *combats* disease with *batteries* of tests and *arsenals* of drugs. And
young staff physicians are still called house *officers.*"[6] And these wars are
fought, of course, for patients.

The push for hard efficiency won't abate easily. Even if unnecessary procedures are better identified and curtailed, eradicating them is only a one-
time saving.[7] All historical trends point to continued growth in doubts about
whether any and all care that serves the medical need of the patient is worth
the money it costs. Randomized clinical trials will be telling more, not less,
about the touch-and-go margins of effective care—what might possibly do a
patient some good but is statistically and economically a dubious bargain.
Both the range of options provided by medical technology and the age of the
population will continue to increase faster than per capita income. Health-
care pressures on government and business budgets will grow, not diminish.[8]

The lines of the continuing prospective debate may thus seem drawn
already. Shouldn't we come clean in our ethics and either honestly sacrifice

commitment to the individual patient or frankly relent in the push for efficiency? Yet such a choice is bleak; we will swallow neither option without a moral gasp.

I propose instead that we reevaluate the conflict itself. Maybe we can avoid having to abandon either side, or perhaps we can at least reduce the force of their collision. I will defend such an ameliorating conception of the conflict. If I am correct, clinicians should be able to keep their oath of commitment to patients while at the same time taking much of larger economic efficiency to heart.

This chapter first critically reviews some of the main proposals for resolving the conflict, explaining their deficiencies and noting the assumption they generally share that genuine commitment to the individual patient stands in unalterable opposition to wider efficiency. I will then describe a way of thinking about rationing labeled *prior consent,* explaining how it greatly softens the conflict and why it is generally more defensible. Finally, I will ward off some likely specific misperceptions of prior consent and extol some of its subtler virtues as a framework for ethically rationing medicine.

Solutions That Fail

Spend Whatever Is Necessary

On one extreme lies the plain denial that overall efficiency has any proper role in medical practice: we should spend whatever is necessary for effective care of the patient, regardless of its cost. The only legitimate cost-containment strategy is to detect and curtail care that does no real good for the patient.[9]

I doubt if any such view that simply rejects one side of the conflict can provide any real resolution. Why should our attraction to efficiency just disappear if we straighten out our medical-ethical thinking? At bottom, spending whatever is necessary simply fails to come to grips with the moral impetus behind efficiency. Economist Williams seems completely correct: it would be fanatical, not ethical, to believe that we must help one person consume resources no matter how small the benefit for him or her, while ignoring other more valuable uses.

Separate Roles

One step toward accommodating economic efficiency would be to separate it from the professional role of practitioners. Society—other people, at earlier stages—must do the rationing of resources. Robert Veatch, for example, claims that asking physicians to do administrators', politicians', and society's job of making rationing decisions is asking them "to remove the Hippocratic Oath from their waiting room walls and replace it with a sign that reads, 'Warning all ye who enter here. I will generally work for your rights and welfare, but if benefits to you are marginal and costs are great, I will abandon you in order to protect society.'"[10] The more carefully administrators, politicians, citizens, and patients control facilities, personnel training, technology development, and insurance coverage policies, the less often individual health-care practitioners will need to make any rationing decisions themselves.[11] Clinicians' practice will then be tightly bounded by whatever rationing policies are handed down to them, but then their own decisions can be governed solely by commitment to the patient.

The strict version of this view holds that it is not enough that practitioners separate their clinical roles from any nonclinical influence they might have in actively formulating rationing policy. They will still be involved too much in rationing if they have any "outside" role in formulating the policies they clinically apply.[12] The looser version of this view, however, would permit them the role of outside consulting about rationing and would only stress their exclusive commitment to individual patients while directly relating to them. The British Medical Association, for example, endorses the physician's duty to "advise" the National Health Service on the equitable and efficient allocation of resources, adding that "this duty is subordinate to his professional duty to the individual who seeks his clinical advice."[13]

In either its loose or its strict version the primary attraction of the separate roles view is to keep both commitment to patient and wider efficiency simultaneously alive. But the attempt is highly problematic. It hardly succeeds in eliminating the basic tension within a practitioner's life. Suppose even that the substantive rationing decisions passed on from "higher" outside levels are so finely tuned that they can simply be applied by the clinician without using judgment to fill in gaps and ambiguities. Wouldn't the clinician still feel conflict in implementing these instructions while professing full commitment to the patient? Implementing rationing decisions would still be the clinician's professional action face to face with patients. How could simply labeling these as different roles remove the essential problem for the one professional person?

In any case, how wise or realistic would it be to fine-tune earlier rationing decisions to the degree that this solution requires? Any given technology will involve a range of potential benefits for different patients. Any disease category will contain a range of different prognoses. Any patient category—age is a perfect example—will contain similar variations. It is simply impossible to sharpen rationing policies enough to pick out the set of treatments, diseases, and people for whom marginal benefits are as great as opportunity costs. If we think of the inevitably crude policy decisions as hard and fast instructional kits for clinicians, we will be prevented from treating in some actual cases where the treatment's benefit is actually worth its cost—for example, not being allowed to prescribe kidney dialysis for a model seventy-year-old with no other problems. Admittedly, dialyzing patients older than sixty-five may generally be inefficient, but if we deny treatment in this particular case, efficiency-motivated rationing will have partially defeated itself. Here both individual patient welfare and larger efficiency favor treatment.[14]

On the other hand, suppose we see our prior rationing policies as looser guidelines. They block out categories of cases as not warranting treatment, but those categories really only alert clinicians to the caution required in exercising their own sense of whether the likely benefits are worth the costs. This probably has significant human welfare advantages over the stricter conception of rationing policies, but it puts us squarely back in the lap of our basic dilemma: providers face to face with patients will be doing active, substantive rationing.

The separate roles view, then, fails to resolve the dilemma. It leaves much of the clinician's conflict between hard efficiency and patient commitment unresolved, and it may even be self-defeating in terms of the very efficiency that led to rationing in the first place.

Justice First

Daniels has given an appealing explanation of why it is so hard for American providers to say no to marginal health care.[15] In the British National Health Service, saying no to marginally beneficial care meets three conditions. First, the opportunity costs of using a treatment are clear; with a fixed annual budget, treating one patient really does mean forgoing benefits for someone somewhere else in the system. Second, systemwide rationing decisions aim at a larger fairness, so it seems unfair to use a treatment on a particular patient outside the lines of those decisions. Third, when practitioners do deny care, they seldom have a conflict of interest—a profit motive—in doing so.[16]

Normally in the United States, at least one of these conditions is missing, and often all are. They are missing at all levels—clinical, institutional, regional, national, and insurance company. The economic incentives in most current U.S. cost-containment measures are not an adequate "substitute for social decisions about health care priorities and the just design of health care institutions."[17]

In practice the justice first view and the separate roles view may look similar, but their reasoning is essentially different. The separate roles approach allegedly resolves the conflict by making practitioners no longer the active rationers. The justice first approach does not necessarily do that. It only claims that for rationing to be acceptable to patients and the public, it must be fair, required by real opportunity costs, and not implemented for the clinician's own gain.

This sounds right. In a profession trusted so much by clients, nothing is more important than fairness and the avoidance of conflict of interest. Upon closer examination, however, justice first is not an adequate conceptual solution of the basic conflict.

Daniels keeps noting the opportunity costs of sacrificing other people's health care, but why must we cite those to justify passing up some beneficial services for an insured patient? Why couldn't opportunity costs of other sorts—fewer non-health-care goods, maybe even fewer for this patient—persuade us equally to pass up some marginal health care? Moreover, the opportunity costs and fairness conditions of the justice first approach require some universal pool of potential patients and some budgetary cap in financing their care, but what if we have independent reasons for allowing somewhat selective pooling or using some other financing scheme than a budgetary cap? In any case, just because Daniels's societywide fairness does not happen to be achievable at this time in our society, why should we throw up our hands and do nothing to restrict marginal care?

The fact that Daniels's initial clue for resolving this conflict is a comparison with Great Britain may also lead to doubt about its success. By no means is the basic moral conflict resolved. Instead of "commitment to the patient," the British speak of "clinical freedom" and "the right of the doctor to act as he thinks is best for an individual patient," but for the practitioner these represent the same essential conflict with efficiency.[18] One bit of evidence that these phrases are not merely pious references is the extreme length to which some British clinicians apparently go when they may not prescribe some treatment for a certain category of patients. To avoid the conflict with efficiency, they will deny, for example, that renal dialysis would do any good for an elderly patient.[19] Such denial often amounts to willing deception of the patient or a slide in standards of care. If clinicians within a national health service that meets Daniels's conditions will go to that length to preserve the face of commitment to the individual welfare of the patient, we might doubt that those conditions satisfactorily resolve the conflict. A health-care system in which Daniels's three conditions are met might be better on other counts than the current American one, but they do not by themselves resolve the basic conflict between patient and society.

Practice Managers

Alan Williams has claimed that physicians have never regarded rationing for hard efficiency as morally intolerable.[20] They have always proudly been practice managers, allocating time among therapeutic practice, learning, teaching, and research. In so doing they have not by any means always acted for the benefit of each of their patients. They impose real sacrifices on some so that others—usually future ones—might benefit. Thus, despite profession of commitment to each patient, physicians themselves have not really regarded the allocation of scarce resources among patients as unethical.

All of this has enormous bite in the current discussion. If it is permissible for physicians to do less in allocating their time than they might for their current patients in order that others might benefit, why should they not be permitted to act that way in using other resources as well? What could be the relevant difference? It is only a small step, then, from traditional medical practice to the allocation of resources for societywide, hard efficiency. The apparent unqualified commitment to each individual patient is only a thin veneer on a quite different, long-standing professional ethic.

This descriptive picture of proper medical practice seems realistic, but the implication that Williams claims can be drawn from it cannot be. Traditional-minded physicians could simply say that their obligation is to take only as many patients as still allows time for the learning, teaching, and research that will not impose sacrifices on any one of them. Even in a capitation payment system such as that for primary care in Britain, doctors are obligated to resist the desire for higher income that could be achieved by adding more patients to their rolls. On both sides of the Atlantic, clinicians are obligated not to oversize their clientele.

Of course, they engage in the appearance of rationing in turning down some patients to keep their loads manageable. But even then they could claim that *they* are not ultimately rationing medicine; it is *society's* obligation to train enough doctors to meet demand. Admittedly providers take holidays, play with their children, and so on, with undoubtedly some negative impact on their patients. But that, too, is hardly rationing resources among patients or denying them even some small possibility of benefit if society trains enough doctors.

Thus, we cannot simply read off of the existing sense of proper practice management any ethical acceptance of imposing sacrifices on some patients to gain greater benefits elsewhere.

The Prior Consent of Patients as Persons

Spending whatever is necessary, separate roles, and justice first share a common conception of the conflict itself. All three views suppose that it is not significantly the individual patient but society—other people, all people—who is protected by efficient rationing.[21] And they think of commitment to the patient in terms of maximizing the welfare of individual patients in their current state of affairs, needing medical help. If these are correct interpretations of the nature of the conflict, it will indeed be difficult to resolve.[22]

But both are misconceptions. What if the hard efficiency side of the conflict represented the individual's own demands even when this results in withholding something of immediate value to the patient? And what if commitment to the individual involved much more than maximizing the welfare of people as *patients?* We would have a much softer conflict on our hands.

This is where the promising line of analysis lies. The point that provides a solution is essentially simple: if individual patients beforehand would have granted consent to the rationing policies and procedures in question (or more clearly yet, if they actually have consented to them), then the appeal of those policies and procedures will rest not merely on attachment to the morally controversial goal of overall aggregate welfare, "efficiency"; such policies will gain their moral force from respecting individual patients' own will.

I shall call this the *prior consent* model for resolving the original conflict. Let's look at three sorts of situations in which consent might be given, with sufficient moral force to justify selective rationing.

The Actual Consent of Subscribers[23]

Suppose that members of a voluntary, cooperative prepaid health plan explicitly consider coverage for a particular treatment, such as adult liver transplants.[24] After surveying the membership and a variety of discussions at different levels, the plan decides not to cover them. At a cost of nearly $300,000 per transplanted patient in first-year care and $6,000 to $7,000 per year per patient for follow-up costs, and with a five-year survival rate of 65 percent, in effect this is a decision that $600,000 could be better spent on other things than five- to twenty-year additional life spans. The decision is publicized to the plan's current and prospective members, and some other plans that cover this procedure are available in the community. Under these circumstances, who would really want to argue that the plan's doctors and nurses are violating their moral oath to patients if they subsequently cooperate with this decision?

To be sure, it is ill patients, not relatively healthy subscribers, with whom those doctors and nurses still finally sit face to face. So some will continue to object: why should we take as our reference point that to which these people have consented at a quite different, earlier point in time? The question is appropriate, but there are answers.

Given the dynamics of the modern health-care economy, the point of subscribing to insurance is the most effective point for people to take control over the scarce resources of their lives. Once patients are insured, whether in private or public arrangements, patients and providers together have strong, natural incentives to overuse care and underestimate opportunity costs. Why not address the problem of controlling the use of care in the face of these incentives at the point in the decision process—insuring—where the essential trouble starts? Sometimes there are reasons for not allowing people to precommit themselves to things they might later want to reject. But the best reason— that a later decision is likely to be better[25]—simply does not hold in health-care rationing contexts. In the later perspective of insured and ill patients, their capacity to control the resources of their larger lives is sharply diminished. Either as communities or as individuals or both, patients want to retrieve that control.

In recent decades the traditional ethic of health care has moved away from paternalistic protection of the patient's welfare toward respect for autonomy. Morally, why should that have happened? Autonomy itself matters because we want to respect the whole person, not just because of some particular circumstance of medical need that people find themselves in at the time.[26] An ethic that ignored the power to choose at an earlier point in time to exercise control over what people know are likely to be their later desires as patients would hardly respect their autonomy as persons in any full or mature sense.

It is entirely possible, of course, that some people at the earlier point of subscribing or voting might choose an open-ended, nonrationing arrangement despite its predicted expense. But even they make that basic judgment from a prior vantage point. There is no other way for them to have much control over the resources of their lives.

The Presumed Consent of Pretreatment Patients

Because the rationing that puts clinicians in a moral corner is by definition not currently in the interest of the patient, we are unlikely to find cases in which patients consent to restrictions on their care. We do find virtually just that, however, in a few cases in which patients would clearly vote for a care-denying, cost-containing policy immediately prior to their care.

A striking, real case of this involves the use of temporary artificial hearts to tide transplant candidates over until a suitably matched donor becomes available. George Annas has pointed out that any transplant surgeon in such a case needs to take account of a crucial fact: with a marked shortage of donor organs, any heart the surgeon might procure for the patient will almost certainly displace another transplant candidate on the waiting list.[27] Temporary heart implants seldom have any net lifesaving effect; they only shift the life saved by the eventual transplant from one person to another, usually at considerable extra expense.

Imagine a group of informed potential transplant recipients considering all of this. Their hearts are already acutely failing, but they would still see themselves as no worse off if transplant surgeons were prevented from indulging in any fantasy of real lifesaving by temporary implant. The question is not what potential transplant recipients would prefer at the point where they knew already that they in particular were being considered for tiding over by artificial implant. We are wondering what policy would be opted for by patients simply awaiting transplant. None of them would be able to hazard any intelligent guess about whether they would end up being saved by use of the implant or left to languish and die without a transplant because supply thereby turned up one organ too short. If they understood all this, including the extra total expense of using temporary implants with no net lifesaving impact, how many would still vote for using temporary implants?

May providers not then presume their informed prior consent to restricting this procedure? Suppose providers ignored their clear, though hypothetical, consent to a policy of passing over artificial implants. Could they defend themselves merely by noting that these patients have not actually consented to such a policy? They might, of course, be blamed for not having asked somehow at the pretreatment stage, if that were feasible. But if that was not feasible—or though if perhaps it was, providers in fact just have not asked—would they not make matters worse by ignoring the fact that very likely they would have consented? The real ethical difficulty in looking to their hypothetical consent has nothing to do with any presuming of their consent per se but only with the degree to which it might not be clear that they would have consented. If providers are really just guessing, admittedly they should not act as if they have patients' consent. (This is discussed further in Chapter 2.)

The Presumed Consent of Subscribers

Suppose, though, that subscribers have not actually consented to restricting care and that there is no immediately pretreatment point at which people would clearly have consented. Any consent to an efficient care-restricting policy would have to be presumed, and only from an earlier point in time. May providers still, just as in the previous immediately pretreatment case, act on people's presumed consent?

Here again many of the same things need to be noted. Providers might be criticized, for instance, for not having asked people for their consent to a rationing decision back at the earlier time of subscribing or voting. Still, if for whatever reasons, good or bad, they have not asked and it is reasonably clear that patients would have consented to a care-restricting policy if they had been, would providers not be making matters worse by plowing on ahead and ignoring the consent they would have given? Again, does not the main ethical difficulty arise only because providers often remain in the dark about whether in fact subscribers would have consented? The questionable aspect is not presumption itself.

One must be careful, of course, about human frailties in consenting to something beforehand. In actual prior consent, subscribers must take thorough account of their possible later situations as patients; likewise, when one is thinking about any of their consent that one might presume, one must think of them as taking that into account. Just as one is reasoning crudely if one attends merely to the immediate patient's desires, so one is also thinking crudely if one discerns policy in earlier points of preference marked by scant understanding of the odds or realities of potential later health crises.

For presumed consent, of course, there will always remain the difficult task of ascertaining what restrictions and procedures would be adopted from the position of imaginative, informed subscribers. It is entirely possible that many rationing questions will be left open when we try to look at them rationally from that earlier point of view. But this, too, can be revealing for thinking out rationing policies. Returning to the basic issue in the separate roles proposal, for example, should practitioners take any active part in decisions to ration? If a person were now deciding to subscribe to a plan, what would he or she say about this?

Suppose the incentives for clinicians to go short on a patient's care for their own financial gain have been minimized by the way they are paid, and the benefits and opportunity costs of many treatments seem to vary widely by circumstance and patient. The patient might then grant a good deal of rationing discretion to clinicians.[28] On the other hand, nurses and physicians may often be surprisingly poor judges of the likely cost-effectiveness ratios of the therapies they use, even though they are very good at ranking their patients' initial needs. Then a patient may hesitate to place any major rationing responsibility on them. Above all it would be unethical for clinicians to take that rationing role on themselves if their prospective patients expected them not to.[29] Equally clearly, however, would it not be permissible for them to take it on if patients expected that they should? Intermediate cases might remain notoriously unclear. What if patients did not expect them *not* to take on this role, for example, but also did not expect them *to* take it on?

In light of such open questions, in fact, maybe what is needed to shape moral standards is simply some help from subscribers. Ideally, here precisely is one of those points on which subscribers should form some expectations. The problem should be seen to fall on them, not primarily on others trying to ascertain in a virtual vacuum what their consent would have been. They need to consider certain prior questions. What is the structure of the plan they are entering or the public program on which the representatives they are electing will vote? To what extent will their clinicians be making decisions to restrict care on the basis of larger efficiency considerations? Is that acceptable to them? Do the financial incentives for clinicians adequately protect them in no-saying situations? (Subscribers might then lean strongly, for example, toward paying physicians by salary rather than fee for service or capitation.)

We can sum up the essential matter of the whole prior consent model more concretely. In a British context, an NHS physician wonders whether she can in good conscience fail to prescribe kidney dialysis, for example, to a patient who will gain several years of problematic life from this expensive technology. The whole NHS decision-making procedure has shaken down to a discernibly short supply of dialysis, and voters have not been about to overturn this by throwing out the NHS "rascals" deemed responsible. Is this physician violating her commitment to her patient if she does not bend the de facto criteria to get the patient on dialysis? As a voter, the patient probably supported the government's policy—at least before his kidney failed, and in any case he supports the political procedures by which those decisions are made. Is not the physician's commitment to him a commitment to a whole person, voter and citizen as well as patient? In fact, would she not be insulting him as an average British citizen proud of his NHS if she ignored scarcity criteria and got him on dialysis?

The details may be different in the American context, but essentially the same principles hold. If a patient has chosen a plan that makes no bones about the fact that times are tough and its staff will occasionally not prescribe all beneficial care, would a clinician not be morally shortsighted and parochial if he saw this person only as a patient needing care? Some questions, to be sure, are more bothersome here than in the British context. Has the person really had a choice of plans with any remotely sufficient information on which to base that choice? But then again, some are less bothersome. Except in Medicare and Medicaid, the difficult questions of political authority do not arise.

For the guideline-setting bureaucrat, the British provider, or the American provider, the relevant question is the same: have these patients consented, or would they have, to the sort of policy restriction now being imposed on them? Focusing on this question will not automatically eliminate the conflict between efficient resource allocation and fidelity to individual patients, but it opens the door to genuine dialogue and possible resolution.

Objections and Advantages

The prior consent model for selectively reconciling hard efficiency with loyalty to patients has further advantages. It can persuasively avoid or refute important common objections to rationing.

The Slide Toward Utilitarianism

One reason people resist rationing is the perception that it can only be justified by a general ethic of maximizing the aggregate utility in society—utilitarianism. If, in turn, a general utilitarian ethic swallows up the fundamental dignity and individuality of persons in a sea of nameless, aggregate well-being, so much for rationing.[30]

Whether or not this characterization of utilitarianism is correct, its identification with rationing is simply mistaken. The prior consent model, for example, if it can provide the justification of rationing, does not aggregate utilities in any such individual-obliterating way. The moral foundation of selective rationing policies insofar as they are endorsed by subscribers or voters is not aggregative welfare per se but autonomy.

Because of this, prior consent can cleanly and easily block the slide toward some of the well-known criticisms that utilitarianism violates individual rights. Consider the issue of killing a person to extract vital organs and save four or five other people by transplant (two kidneys, a heart, a liver, and a pancreas). Modified in a certain way, this becomes the so-called survival lottery: one person is selected by lot and forced to be the donor-victim.[31] Its justification is, first, that it would raise average life expectancy and, second, that since no one could tell beforehand that he or she would turn out to be the unlucky conscript, everyone would find it in his or her interest to consent to such an arrangement. Yet if our considered, stubborn intuitions still object to such a lottery, does that not throw both utility and prior consent into moral doubt?

The argument founders, however, on a central point: are people so concerned about the shortage of donor organs given their possible need for a transplant that they really would consent to such a live dissection lottery? I doubt it. Utility may endorse a survival lottery, but consent almost certainly does not.[32]

Equity and Justice

Rationing for greater efficiency, will we not end up unfairly slighting those who are so poorly situated in their health from the start that much of their care produces little benefit though it is the only chance they have?

This fear forgets the precise nature of the relationship between consent and efficiency. The prior consent model for thinking about rationing does not endorse any and every gain in efficiency. For a distinctly disadvantaged individual, if one can discern no point in that person's life at which he or she would have consented to the restriction that now ends up denying care, a whole army of other people's consent cannot by itself justify applying that restriction to him or her.[33] Far from ignoring the claims of especially disadvantaged individuals, prior consent leans in the opposite direction, giving the genuine, long-run equity claims of individuals virtual veto power over efficiency considerations. Someone who comes to the issue of whether or not to consent to rationing policy already knowing his or her illness need not be exposed to the same limitations on costworthy care that the rest of us willingly accept.[34]

This also reveals that prior consent is not a cover for some kind of fundamental ethical individualism. The prior consent model's initial, unstated assumption is right in line with mainstream convictions about the communal importance of medical care: social justice does not allow us to brush off the cosmic misfortunes of accident and disease and leave people without assistance. It is precisely because social justice calls us to help our fellow human beings in situations of injury and illness that we find ourselves in such moral consternation when trying to put limits on the care that might help. The consent of the individual subscriber or citizen only comes into play to limit our obligation to provide assistance after our sense of justice has created and nurtured that obligation to start. Consent does not work in a moral vacuum.[35]

The Worth of Different Persons

To most people rationing connotes trading off one person's care for another's. That, in turn, seems to imply that one person's very life is worth more than another's. Some states of existence may be more or less worth living than others, but should we compare the very value of persons themselves?

The objection voices something very important, but it simply does not work against rationing health care according to patients' own prior consent.

The crucial reason why Mary gets dialysis and Harry does not is not that any of us has judged him to be worth less than her. It is that Harry himself has endorsed the decision that her sort of life should be saved before his. He may not do that at the time of treatment, and he has probably not ever explicitly endorsed such a decision, but for rationing to be justified the procedures or criteria by which his own life ends up now being judged worth less than Mary's must be in some sense his own. Without that, prior consent has not justified any rationing at all; with it, it has justified rationing with individuals' own judgments about the relative worth of saving their lives.[36]

Hardened Hearts

One observer has been quoted as saying that physicians in Great Britain are at first "appalled" at letting treatable kidney dialysis patients die, but then, like "good Germans . . . they learn to stomach it." They are not burdened with guilt and do not struggle with their compassion; they just "harden their hearts," eased by their own myth that "little of real benefit" can be done.[37]

Such cover-up is terribly disturbing. But note that the tendency for it to occur is greater the sharper one draws the conflict between hard efficiency and commitment to the patient. Without any moral connection between concern for this person-patient and efficient rationing, how can one blame sensitive providers for defensively reacting by hardening their real moral hearts? The dependable way around this danger is to conceive of rationing right at the start as something done without moral abandonment of the patient. This would be the practice of strong medicine, but it would be neither callous nor insensitive.

No matter how a rationing policy gets justified, if it is justified providers ought to be able to stick by it face to face with patients without losing their compassion. That will be easier the more clearly rationing policies and criteria are grounded in patients' own prior consent.

Deception and Instability

Compromises, not genuine resolutions of this conflict, have the unfortunate result of leaving a terribly uneasy peace. They are much more likely to end up in the kind of deception that critics of rationing are fond of citing—for example, in the British policy of rarely giving renal dialysis to anyone older than sixty-five. Clinicians are supposed to be committed to their patients; if that commitment is really compromised by rationing policies they have to carry out, they will naturally want to tell patients who are denied life-prolonging treatment only that there is little that can be done for them.

This is not only blatant deception of the patient; it is also a major point of instability in the professional side of any rationing arrangement. Clinicians of integrity will refuse to believe the deception, and some will work hard and with conviction to skirt rationing criteria and get their patients treated. If they adopt the prior consent model's view that they can respect their commitment to their individual patients while selectively restricting some beneficial care, they will surely be less likely to undercut efficient rationing policies.

Of course, even the more basic sort of resolution accomplished by prior consent will be vulnerable to political and emotional disturbances. The acceptance and stability of the prior consent view's interpretation of respect for the patient is ultimately contingent on people's ability to see that there are important points of decision about resource allocation that occur before they become ill patients. At times it will be extremely difficult not only for patients and their families but also for subscribers and citizens to keep those points in mind. Individuals who need particular treatments get wheeled up on state house steps, for example, daring public authorities or insurance companies to let them die for want of coverage.

That is a terribly effective tactic for undermining rationing, but is it legitimate? Prior consent helps us understand why it probably is not. Accurately envisioning the nature of one's potential plight is required of anyone in the prior consent situation, but what happens psychologically when victims are placed in front of the news cameras typically goes far beyond that. The serious, important question for policy formation purposes—would people give prior consent to rationing here or not?—gets washed away in the emotional flood of the immediately pleading individual.

Of all the proposed resolutions of the original conflict, prior consent gives us by far the greatest confidence and ability to stick to our rationing guns in this kind of "public patient" situation. If we understand its selective justification of hard efficiency, we should be able to look patients in the eye with little moral hesitation. It will be hard but hardly disloyal. Rationing is always distasteful medicine to swallow, but it may be just what we, as well as the doctor, ordered.

We must not grasp desperately at just any resolution of the conflict between clinical commitment to patients and the achievement of efficiency. We should also, however, not inflate the conflict into something greater than it is. The "spend whatever is necessary," separate roles, and justice first solutions presume an inflated picture of the conflict itself, and the practice managers approach cannot pull what it claims out of the traditional clinician's ethic. Armed with a reinterpretation of commitment to the individual patient, prior consent is a more productive and persuasive way of thinking about rationing. In cases of actual consent or the close presumed consent of pretreatment patients, the model's moral justification of care-restricting policies is clear and solid. For the more distant presumed consent of subscribers and voters, its argumentative force is less firm. The primary source of doubts there, though, is not consent or its presumption itself but uncertainty about whether informed, imaginative, understanding subscribers would actually have consented.

That uncertainty can be turned into a virtue: prior consent does not give a simple green light to any and all efficient policies. It sometimes tells us itself when those policies are morally problematic. And in cases where it does justify rationing, it achieves the more thorough and stable resolution of the conflict for which we have hoped. It does not push us into the undesirable implications of utilitarianism, it does not ignore equity and justice, and it does not objectionably compare the worth of different persons.

Discriminating providers may ration care with a clean conscience. Even a right-minded economist could take their Hippocratic oath.

NOTES

1. This is the colloquial sense of *Hippocratic oath:* moral loyalty to individual patients. There is much more to be said, of course, about the original oath itself and Hippocrates himself, the corpus of writings and sayings attributed to him, the complex of often antithetical Greek and Judeo-Christian influences on Western medical ethics, and the typically profession-oriented rather than patient-oriented focus of the various versions of the Hippocratic oath. See Kass (1985b), pp. 224–46; Pellegrino (1973); Richards (1973); Veatch (1981), pp. 3–49, 147–69; and Veatch and Mason (1987). At this point I leave undefined just what the oath requires loyalty to. The prominent candidates are maximum welfare (best interests) and autonomy of individual patients. The original oath of Hippocrates seems to focus exclusively on the patient's best interest and presumes that the physician knows what that is.

2. Angell (1985), pp. 1206–7. This view is reiterated in countless places. See, for example, the British oncologist quoted in Aaron and Schwartz (1984), p. 107; Dyer (1986); Morreim (1985), p. 36; and the September 15, 1986, minutes of the Ethics Council of Group Health Cooperative of Puget Sound, p. 6.

3. Thurow (1984), p. 1569.

4. Mooney (1986), pp. 98–100.

5. Williams (1985c), p. 8.

6. Winslow (1984), p. 33.

7. Schwartz (1987). For the contrary view, see Brook and Lohr (1986).

8. Ginzberg (1987).

9. Angell (1985).

10. Veatch (1986), p. 38.

11. Fuchs (1984b), p. 1573; and Levinsky (1984).

12. Veatch and Mooney go the farthest in stating this view. Veatch (1986), p. 38: If physicians are to have any role in rationing decisions beyond conveying medical facts, they

must adopt an ethic of full, societywide beneficence and justice, but as professional clinicians they have no special insights on translating such an ethic into policy. Mooney (1986), p. 125, reacts to the British Medical Association's endorsement of the doctor's "general duty to advise on ... [the] equitable allocation and efficient utilisation" of limited resources within the National Health Service; in the achievement of equity and efficiency "clinicians need to be the advised, not the advisors."

13. British Medical Association (1980), p. 35.

14. This basic problem is posed by Morreim (1987a) and responded to by Veatch (1987). See also Morreim (1988b) and Veatch (1988b).

15. Daniels (1986). Cassel (1985) views the necessary conditions for resolving the problem of rationing as very similar. Generally I will use Daniels's specific statement of the view. I have coined the label *justice first* for the essential position I am using Daniels and Cassel to represent; their published positions may not carry all of my label's connotations.

16. The capitation payment system is used for primary-care providers in the NHS. Actually, capitation still gives physicians an indirect incentive to undertreat patients—not any particular treatment, and certainly not in referring to specialists, but in devoting time to the patient. The less time spent per patient, the more patients a physician can have on his or her rolls.

17. Daniels (1986), p. 1384.

18. Maynard and Ludbrook (1980), p. 29. As they note, reference to clinical freedom was incorporated in the 1944 White Paper preliminary to establishing the NHS.

19. Aaron and Schwartz (1984), p. 101. For an important criticism of Aaron and Schwartz's interpretation of British medical practice, see Miller and Miller (1986).

20. Williams (1985c), especially pp. 5–6.

21. Several people already quoted reveal this. Angell (1985), p. 1206, refers to the two masters: the patient and "society's coffers." Veatch (1986), p. 38, speaks of "abandoning" the patient in order to "protect society."

22. Spending whatever is necessary and the separate roles approach clearly share these assumptions. The justice first view may not do so as much, though it says nothing to emphasize any departure from them. As for the practice managers model, it says that clinicians' ethical commitment is not to individual patients, so that the reconciliation it accomplishes is not with any such commitment to begin with. I propose to reconcile a full commitment to the individual patient with selective hard efficiency.

23. To broaden the application, one would need to speak of voters in a democracy with a national health service, not just subscribers to a private plan. At many points in my argument this can be done, though ultimately such extension will rest on other arguments of political philosophy about a democratic community's control over individual dissent which go far beyond the confines of this book.

24. In something very close to the detail hypothesized here, Group Health Cooperative of Puget Sound considered heart and liver transplants in 1985–86. The outcome of their long and complex process was board of trustees approval of coverage for heart transplants and for liver transplants in children with biliary atresia but not coverage of liver transplants for adults. See Menzel (1988), pp. 157–58.

25. Regan (1983), p. 129; and Thaler (1982), p. 180. Schelling's discussion (1984) is also directly relevant. Although he is sympathetic to binding oneself later by decisions made now, he points out that the law does not generally listen to one's earlier self (p. 96). It enforces contracts with others but not those with oneself. Note that the binding of oneself that occurs in consenting to rationing policies at the point of subscription to a health plan is very much a contract with others for the premium structure and financial integrity of the enterprise.

26. This is roughly the "integrity" view of autonomy taken by Dworkin (1986a).

27. Annas (1985). Any dispute of this factual claim would have to rest on tissue-matching problems. The donor heart, because of matching problems, would have to have been wasted had it not gone to the recipient tided over by the artificial implant.

28. Fleck (1987), p. 2, surmises that in health maintenance organizations, physicians who act as rationing agents are carrying out the wishes of their patients.

29. Brock (1986a), p. 769.

30. This seems to be at the heart of Veatch's criticism of allowing the clinician to make rationing decisions. See Veatch (1986), pp. 37–38.

31. Harris (1975).

32. Some will still think that the example shows prior consent to be fundamentally wrong-headed reasoning: we still might consent to such a lottery, yet we are sure that it would still be a morally objectionable arrangement. But are we so sure at all that if everyone who participated clearly consented to it, it really would be morally objectionable?

33. See Chapter 6 on imperiled newborns for an extended discussion of one such case.

34. This is an immensely complex matter in the case of the more ill as distinct from the less ill. See Menzel (1983), pp. 194–203.

35. My model is thus not easily vulnerable to the charge of individualism that Larry Churchill makes against consent and contract models of medical ethics in his recent book on rationing. Churchill throws this charge around loosely. He labels John Rawls's contractual theory of social justice fundamentally individualistic, for example, simply because it extracts the principles of justice from consent. That ignores the crucial role that intuitions of justice play in Rawls's setting up the "original position" from which contractors work out official principles. See Churchill (1987), especially pp. 44–45.

36. For an extended discussion of this issue, see Chapter 5 on quality-adjusted life years.

37. British observer quoted by Halper (1985), p. 77.

2

Presuming a Patient's Consent to Risk

Doubts and Their Importance

A doctor skeptically wonders, "what is the patient's interest in reducing . . . the aggregate cost of health care by foregoing . . . a CAT scan?"[1] This simple doubt constitutes a powerful moral challenge to rationing medical care in the interest of overall efficiency in the society. In Chapter 1, I argued that there is often a way for health-care providers to extricate themselves from this conflict: their commitment to patients is compatible with rationing their care if they were previously willing to take the risk of having later care withheld. But this willingness is prior to the time of actual, often urgent need, and even then it will seldom have been overtly expressed. The argument has to assume that people may be disadvantaged merely on the basis of a prior consent to risk that they may not have actually, expressly given.

If we look critically at what is going on here, we may wonder whether such an argument requiring this assumption can be even remotely right-headed. Questions immediately arise:

1. If a person only consents to the risk that he or she might need care that will be withheld, has he or she consented to the care actually being withheld? In a disturbing parallel, surely one has not consented to being burglarized simply because one admittedly accepted a greater risk of theft when one chose to buy a house in a higher-crime neighborhood at a somewhat lower price.
2. If it is correctly presumed that a person would have given consent but that person never actually has done so, can anything be done to him or her? Suppose, for example, that someone mysteriously leaves a bottle of wine

on your doorstep, one you frequently buy for five dollars. You are delighted and drink it that night with a friend. You surely aren't obligated to pay if the person who left the wine later demands a bargain-rate three-dollar reimbursement. Yet that person could claim—quite correctly, as a matter of fact—that if you had been asked, you would certainly have agreed to buy it for that price.

Does the very core of the prior consent model for rationing medical care then start to crumble? To preserve the argument, I must explain carefully how presumed prior consent to risk does real moral work. This chapter focuses directly on this more fundamental philosophical part of the argument. I will make my points by a series of specific examples, sometimes medical, and throughout the implications for health care will be made explicit. The basic issue, though, has much wider ramifications. Implicit, presumed, hypothetical consent has not only played an important role in traditional theories of political obligation but is currently central to well-known viewpoints in social policy analysis:

1. In constitutional law, a common-sense response to "strict construction-ism" is to bring founding fathers conceptually up to date via presumed consent, trying to ascertain what sort of wording they would have chosen to convey their ideas had they envisioned future circumstances.[2]
2. The most prominent proponent of "economic analysis of law," a contro-versial view urging that legal decisions be geared to maximize society's total wealth, has spurned the utilitarianism[3] most readers thought was his philosophical parentage. Instead, Richard Posner argues, consent is the "operational basis" of efficiency: "consent to efficient solutions can be presumed."[4]
3. As "cost-benefit analysis" clarifies its philosophical foundations, it has increasingly resorted to hypothetical consent—the consent people would give to trading safety for money, for example. Major proponents of cost-benefit analysis sum up their view by saying that "the government . . . should seek the outcomes that fully informed individuals would choose for themselves if voluntary exchange were feasible."[5]

The list could go on. Presuming people's prior consent has had significant employment in policy analysis. It needs careful defense.

First, though, we should define what the debate is actually about. Virtually everyone thinks that actual consent has greater moral force than presumed hypothetical consent. An explicit natural death directive, for example, gen-erally provides a better reason for withholding life-support measures than if we had to infer what someone would want from the kind of person he or she was. For one thing, people see intrinsic value in making their own explicit choices.[6] The issue, then, is not at all whether presumed prior consent has as much moral force as actual consent—of course it does not. The issue is only how much force it has, if any. The challenge comes from those who claim that even when consent actually would have been forthcoming in hypothetical, envisioned circumstances, virtually none of the value of individual freedom is retained by presumed consent. I will argue to the contrary: something very significant for practical, real-world freedom is lost if we ignore consent simply because it is hypothetical.

This chapter does not ask whether some variety of consent is *necessary* for collectively restricting later choices. That would be to ask whether refusal or absence of consent should constitute a moral veto of collective restrictions. To be sure, the very category of presumed consent is often used to claim unanimous consent for some policy, as if a single refusal would constitute a veto. And undoubtedly, if presumed consent counts in moral arguments, presumed refusal of consent should also count for something. But for how much? Refusal of consent might be outweighed by other moral considerations— whether it is is not our concern here.

The issue is also not whether it is proper to refer to highly idealized versions of consent. The question is whether the consent that particular real people would in fact have previously given can substitute for the actual consent that is regarded as morally justifying a given measure. This is a kind of hypothetical consent, but it avoids the telling query to which any consent of hypothetical persons is vulnerable: why is there "any good reason to be bound by deals that might be reached by somebody who wasn't me"?[7] Furthermore, one may hold people to no higher qualifying conditions of rationality in talking about whether they would have consented than one holds them to in their actual consent. However few or many irrationalities of real people are acceptable in actual consent, exactly those could also be acceptable in presumed consent—no more, no fewer.

Comparisons with Consent: Compensation

When economists want to relate the value of efficiency to consent, they will often talk about compensation. They start by defining a state as *Pareto superior* to another if at least one person is better off than she would be in the other state and no one is worse off. This is largely why free exchanges occur— with exchange, people move to a Pareto-superior situation in which no one is worse off.

In itself, Pareto superiority is a relatively uninteresting notion. For controversial social situations, it hardly ever holds; any substantive change will make someone worse. Pareto relationships get interesting only with an important modification. A change is *potential* Pareto superior if some persons gain enough to be able to compensate all the losers and still leave everyone better off.[8] Presumably this is precisely what happens in any move to a more efficient situation; if the winners cannot compensate the losers to leave everyone better off, the move is simply not efficient.

A whole torrent of objections, however, can be raised against whatever moral force potential Pareto superiority might be thought to have. Imagine the following:

1. Factory A saves so much money by not installing pollution control equipment that it could then compensate neighboring homeowners who are adversely affected more than what clean air is worth to them, and still be better off itself.

If the homeowners are the only ones affected, polluting rather than controlling is here the efficient, welfare-maximizing course of action. Since the compensation to them is only potential, however, and not actually paid, few would put much moral stock in the bare fact that failing to install pollution control equipment was efficient. Unless the losing homeowners actually get compensated, no one is impressed.

Another example appears to be parallel but is importantly different:

2. Factory B relocates. The new town's residents gain enough that they could compensate the residents of the former town for more than their losses and still be better off themselves.

Even if compensation is not actually paid, more can be said here in defense of Factory B's relocation than in defense of Factory A's uncompensated pollution. In both cases a factory's behavior increases overall utility. Utility alone, however, gives Factory A no green light, for the homeowners around it can very plausibly claim to have existing moral rights not to have their property actively and knowingly harmed. By contrast any alleged rights of the former town's residents to employment at Factory B are more dubious, so consent or compensation is not so clearly needed to allow efficiency its moral pull.

Thus, if preexisting moral rights are present, merely potential Pareto superiority (efficiency) controls little by itself. Either actual compensation or some sort of consent is required.[9] This holds for efficiency in medicine as well as for efficiency anywhere else. It is thus clearly understandable how, in the individually urgent and injustice-of-illness context of common medical situations, we are inclined to demand some sort of actual compensation or consent before we give efficiency much weight.

So much for potential compensation. What about actual compensation of those who lose? It might appear that this would carry much more weight, but without some kind of consent it, too, has little moral force. Consider the following:

> 3. Factory C pollutes its neighboring homeowners, lowering their housing values. It doesn't compensate them anew, however, for a hidden compensation has already been made. They initially bought their houses at the lower prices created by the fear that the factory's growing pollution might eventually depress housing values.

How is this a case of equivalent compensation? An obvious test comes to mind. If the homeowners had clearly understood (1) the drop in housing values that would occur if Factory C polluted at this level, (2) the probability that its pollution would grow to such a damaging level, and (3) the immediate gains they would already realize in buying a home there at already depressed prices, would they have actually agreed to buy their houses there in the first place? We are back to prior consent as the crucial condition.

One might think that current or subsequent compensation would fare better than this prior kind. But it, too, fares no better unless connected to some sort of consent.

> 4. A rapist immediately compensates his victim. The victim has neither actually nor presumably consented to any sexual act.

If the victim had actually freely consented beforehand, the act would either be seduction or, if for monetary compensation, prostitution. The case here is different; the victim has not consented.

"Adequate" compensation is itself puzzling in this case. How would we determine what was adequate? If we compute that from what the victim would have been willing to pay to reduce only a significant risk of being raped, "adequacy" would reflect only the victim's consent to the risk of rape, not to the rape itself. It still would not be compensation equivalent to the harm she has now actually experienced. For this we might think for a moment that her hypothetical prostitution price might be a more appropriate reference point—it involves a known outcome, not just a risk. But it will not remotely do, either, for it entirely omits the force and terror of rape. Probably no notion of adequate compensation is possibly coherent here.

More importantly, even if we could somehow conceptualize the adequacy of compensation, it would hardly legitimize the rapist's behavior. Criminals do not get white hats if only they toss enough cash at their victims as they barge through life.

The moral limitations of actual compensation compared to consent are revealed by another case, this time a real one:

> 5. A negligent surgeon performs contraceptive surgery on mother who subsequently bears a normal child. The parents sue for compensation, but they acknowledge that because the surprise joys of parenting have already exceeded their burdens in having an additional child, they have suffered no net harm from the mistake.[10]

It is plausible to doubt whether a court should award the parents legal compensation from the negligent physician, especially if the jurisdiction is one in which punitive damages are generally not allowed in civil suits. But one thing is clear: the actual compensation that may have already taken place does not take the physician off the moral hook. The parents' rights of consent in having children have been violated, though their welfare may not have been decreased.

The conclusion seems clear. What it is right for us to do to others is determined more fundamentally by people's consent than by whether we adequately compensate them. Both actual compensation and the economist's surrogate for efficiency, potential compensation, gain what moral permission-creating power they might have from the hypothetical prior consent they can sometimes elicit.

Consent to Risk

So we come to consent itself. We must first clarify several things about consenting to risk.

> 6. A home buyer has two houses to choose from. The first costs less but is in a higher-crime neighborhood. The second, in a safer area, costs more. The buyer weighs these comparative advantages, buys the first house, then gets burglarized.

The home buyer was apparently equivalently compensated for the risk he took by a lower purchase price or he would not have made the purchase. He clearly agreed to take the risk of burglary.[11] But note that this gives no moral permission whatsoever to the burglary. One critic, Jules Coleman, sees this example as demonstrating that prior consent can legitimize harms and losses no more than compensation can.[12]

Yet that use of this example reflects important confusions. In this case the home buyer consented only to the risk of being burglarized, not to the burglary itself.[13] The same is true of almost any consent-to-risk situation.

> 7. A lottery player spends $10, willing to take the 99,999-in-100,000 chance of losing in order to have the 1-in-100,000 chance of winning $1 million. The lottery player loses.

We naturally talk about this as a case in which the lottery player consented to "lose $10," but technically she did not. She consented only to the fair drawing of lots in which she would very probably lose. This is shown by what is sure to be her reaction if some of the number slips were, say, stuck together so that hers had no chance of being drawn.

This point applies directly to restricting medical care. Suppose a person consents beforehand to a policy of not providing hemodialysis for people older than seventy; then, at age seventy, this person's kidneys fail. Has he consented to dying at age seventy from lack of dialysis? Not really. Precisely what nurses and doctors may balk at in using a prior consent model to reconcile their patient commitment with denial of care is that it seems incredibly contrived for them to look a patient in the eye and construe that what he or she has done in earlier risk taking was consent to actually dying now for lack of care. This seems contrived because it *is* contrived. The patient has not consented to any such thing at all, only to taking a certain relatively low risk of dying from lack of dialysis. If it were revealed, for example, that all along the patient's kidneys had actually had an extremely high chance of failing (and that there was some very feasible way by which he could have known that), he would surely rebel at now being denied dialysis on the pretext that he had previously consented. (Patient preceptions of fate connect here with patient anger. If the patient's kidneys were already destined to fail at the time he took the risk of being left without dialysis, he might feel something was unfair about now holding him to the risk he earlier agreed to take. The feeling is understandable, of course, but assuming that no one was in a position to have known then what fate had already decreed, this can hardly constitute any objection.)

Note that in the homebuying-burglary case, consent legitimizes only letting the risk of burglary stand; it does not sanction the burglary itself. This is also true of the typical lottery loser: losing per se is not what becomes right. One's consent only removes any obligation people might have to reduce one's risk of losing $10, so one has no complaint against anyone when one loses.[14] Similarly, in the burglary case, the home buyer has no complaint against the police for not extending themselves beyond the level of protection he had every good reason to expect they would provide.

Furthermore, burglars are different from most people who are parties to the occurrence of losses and harms. They can stop the harm, but not only that, we already know that they unquestionably ought to have stopped it. In the risk cases in which consent does carry weight, there simply is no one of whom those things can be said. In most cases of rationing medical care, for example, precisely what consent is being used to decide is the open question of whether someone ought to have reduced the risk.

A major point about morally relevant consent is also involved in these consent and risk examples. Consent must be free and uncoerced. One analysis— we might call it the rights view—says that a choice is coerced if the alternative with which one is presented is itself already viewed as a violation of one's rights. For example, the choice to hand over money to a robber who points a gun at one's head is not free because the alternative—being shot—is clearly regarded as a violation of one's rights. But the alternative when one previously chose a policy of excluding care that now turns out to be one's life support was only paying more in premiums or taxes for fuller coverage. On most views that is hardly any violation of one's rights.

In rationing care we need to keep these important aspects of prior consent to risk in mind. Usually consent is to the risk of harm, not to the harm itself. When it is to risk of harmful denial of care, uncoerced consent helps to morally legitimize denial in only one respect: people have no complaint when care is harmfully denied unless that is something already, independently regarded as wrong.

Presumed Prior Consent

How much of any of this will change if prior consent has not actually been given but would have been given if people had had a chance to mull matters over? A family of examples about the principle of fairness (or the duty of fair play) is closely related.[15] One famous example is from Nozick:

> 8. A citizen cannot avoid receiving the benefits of a cooperative public address system that broadcasts to her community of 365 people. Her annual share of the system's programming takes a day of her time. To her the system's benefits are worth that expense, but she has never consented to the arrangement. Others contribute their day.[16]

Is this person obligated by fairness to contribute? Nozick claims that she is not, even when her benefits from the operation exceed her proportion of its costs. Other uses of her time may have been even more profitable, and even if this was as beneficial a use of time for her as any other, and even if she therefore would presumably have consented to create this operation, an obligation of fairness to contribute is dubious unless she has actually consented.[17]

One point regarding the principle of fairness directly relates to presumed prior consent. Unless we are dealing with public goods that everyone wants regardless of their particular individual desires, mere receipt of benefits without some element of volitional acceptance seems morally impotent.[18] For an obligation to come into existence some element of willfulness must be present: voluntary acceptance of the benefit, participation in the common enterprise, presumed consent, or actual consent. Acceptance of benefits and participation in an enterprise, however, are in principle vague in a way consent is not. Despite the often great evidential difficulty in ascertaining whether one would have consented, what we are looking for is at least conceptually clear: would one have freely and expressly said yes had one been asked? Furthermore, even if acceptance were clarified, it would seem too weak a condition to create fairness obligations. But requiring actual participation or consent would seem to be asking too much. Presumed consent appears to be actual consent's promising cousin for understanding how fairness works.[19]

Just any presumed consent will not work, though. Again one of Nozick's cases, raised more briefly at the beginning of this chapter, is suggestive:

> 9. Someone mysteriously leaves a bottle of wine on your doorstep, one you frequently buy for five dollars. You are pleasantly surprised, check to verify that in fact you did not order it, and proceed to imbibe and enjoy its contents with a friend. The next day, the person who left the wine demands three dollars as reimbursement.[20]

If you had actually been approached, indeed you would have agreed to pay three dollars for the wine. Yet few would ever say that you are now obligated to pay. Here hypothetical consent, despite the fact that it is perfectly correctly estimated, is still morally impotent. Does this not show that presumed consent arguments are in principle wrong-headed?

This example only demonstrates a crucial qualification we all would want to impose on presumed consent arguments. Presumed consent loses its force in the wine-bottle case because the person who left the wine obviously could have approached you to obtain your actual consent to pay three dollars. He could have called you before coming by to leave the bottle or, if circumstances precluded that, at least attached a note when he left it. It was his mistake to ignore these easy avenues to getting your actual consent.[21] Actual consent is still preferable even when it is very clear what that consent would be; for one thing, people see intrinsic value in making their own explicit choices.[22]

Of course, if this intrinsic good of explicit choices is consent's sole value, hypothetical consent will carry no moral weight. But the intrinsic good of explicit choices is not the sole value at stake in this larger business of consent. Bringing decisions in line with one's values and beliefs also plays a major role in creating consent's moral importance. To test this suggestion, imagine examples in which the only consent possible is hypothetical. If a patient is comatose, should the physician simply say, "Well, here there is obviously no intrinsic value any longer in the patient's explicit participation, so I am going to make the decision to keep him alive or not solely on the basis of my own values"? Both in relation to the future if the patient should ever wake up and in relation the value the patient already has in living a life and dying a death that is his own, it is vitally important that the physician consult what the patient would decide if he were conscious. To cut this out of the package of values we refer to as respecting a person's consent would be like taking the seat, handle bars, brakes, and tires off a bicycle and then claiming that since the frame, pedals, and wheels are left, we have only stolen a few incidentals.[23]

The lesson for our troublesome cases is clear: a crucial condition of presuming consent is that obtaining actual consent be either impossible or in some sense prohibitively costly. In the rough sense, "prohibitively costly" simply means what the actual individual, with his or her actual values, would agree is too high a cost for upgrading from presumed to actual consent.[24] In the wine-bottle case, of course, the cost is tiny. This condition may also explain some doubts about the role of presumed consent in the public-address-system case.[25]

There is an equally important qualification on the prior consent part of presumed prior consent arguments.

> 10. At some earlier time a customer actually agreed to buy a widget from a widget maker for the going price then of $100. Since then the bottom has dropped out of the widget market. Citing the customer's presumed prior consent, the widget maker tries to recover $100 in damages for the widget the customer now will not buy.[26]

The widget maker would not and should not win the lawsuit. Any court would be likely to observe that there is all the difference in the world between hypothetical and actual consent.

That difference, however, is explained by something more fundamental. We have already called attention to part of it: in commercial cases such as this, people find it relatively easy to insist on actual contracts. We also have to have some reason for referring back to a prior point in time, for looking back then for the consent we might presume. In many cases there is no reason for doing that. In the widget case, what need did the customer have for insur-

ing against market changes back then and locking the two parties into the
$100 price? Absent special circumstances, there was absolutely no need, so
the widget maker looks utterly silly in suing the customer. To invoke a presumed prior consent argument, we must be able to explain why it is important to refer back to that prior point in time instead of limiting ourselves to
the present.

In this respect restrictions on the use of health care can provide a helpful
contrast:

> 11. A desperate patient, insured by Efficient Care, needs renal dialysis costing
> $30,000 per year. It will likely give her another five years of life, of signifi-
> cantly diminished quality. The patient now thinks this survival is worth
> $30,000 a year, but had she been asked earlier whether people should be
> covered in such circumstances at this cost-benefit ratio, she would undoubt-
> edly have said no.

Suppose that the crucial condition of presumed consent arguments is met:
there is no feasible, non–prohibitively costly way to have approached the
patient and other subscribers for their actual consent to particular possible
restrictions on care such as the one Efficient Care would now like to enforce.
Nothing in the patient's present will justifies restricting dialysis, but all the
facts of her prior willingness to take risks to save money point to her presumable, prior consent to restricting coverage. The most serious question is thus
not about the evidence on the basis of which to extrapolate the patient's prior
consent. It is about whether it is correct in principle to refer to that earlier
point in time.

Unlike the widget case, there is good reason here for saying that the prior
reference point of the insurance subscriber is more correct than that of the
patient in trouble. Confining the cost of health care to that which is truly
worth its benefits is made enormously difficult precisely because we insure
for care. Thereafter neither the patient nor the physician will have much
incentive to forgo care of any possible benefit to the patient regardless of its
cost. Why not, then, address the problem of saying no to dubiously costworthy care in the face of the distorted incentives back at that very point of insurance where the trouble starts? Since the point of subscription is the most effective point at which people can take control over the scarce resources of their
lives, respect for the patient as a whole person allows us to refer back to that
prior point for reading her consent. It may even *demand* that we refer back
to that prior point.

This whole context of managing resources for larger segments of one's life
is missing in some of the examples that give us most serious pause about
using consent from a prior reference point. Take the following case:

12. A Jehovah's Witness yesterday, before he ever needed a blood transfusion, insisted that he never be allowed to have one. Then today, when he needs a transfusion, he completely competently pleads for one, apparently just because he wants so badly to live.[27]

Most people would probably think this patient should be transfused, even knowing that tomorrow he would very likely be as appalled by the transfusion as he was yesterday appalled by its prospect. Yet if the patient would and should be transfused in this case, why should physicians not save the desperate patient who now wants lifesaving dialysis though she had previously consented to a policy of denying that care in what is now her sort of case?[28]

There are important differences. Most importantly, in consenting to a cost-saving policy, the kidney patient has entered into a quasi-contractual cooperative scheme that cannot easily survive if exceptions are allowed after the fact. By contrast, the Jehovah's Witness is involved in an entirely private situation. No implicit or explicit agreement of any kind is necessary to make the institutional arrangements function.

Furthermore (and less critically), it is not clear whether the kidney patient has now really changed her mind fully about the policy to which she previously agreed. Maybe she is just understandably dissenting now because of her bad luck, which would carry little weight in the context of a cooperative scheme. A full change of mind would cause greater concern, but that is not nearly so likely to be what has actually happened. Does she now really think that in managing her and her society's resources over time, a more inclusive (and expensive) policy that covered dialysis in the current circumstances would be best? How can we possibly believe she really thinks that? Maybe the Jehovah's Witness, by contrast, has really changed his mind about the larger importance of his religious belief compared to the value of his earthly life, even if that change is temporary. Despite examples such as the Jehovah's Witness case, prior consent normally takes control in a rationing context.

In justifying the rationing of medical care, then, presuming patients' prior consent to risk is a morally satisfactory substitute for actual consent if we heed important qualifications on its various components:

1. Presumed consent counts for little unless approaching people for their actual consent is impossible or prohibitively costly.
2. There must be important advantages for the sort of case at hand in making decisions at a prior point in time.[29]
3. Consent to risk, whether actual or presumed, does not legitimize a harm itself. It does mean, however, that unless the harm risked is itself a course

of behavior by others that we already assume to be wrong, the person consenting has no complaint if it actually occurs.

4. Generally, any invocation of presumed prior consent carries the burden of accurately discerning what people would in fact have agreed to. It is always a relevant objection to any argument invoking presumed prior consent simply to dispute whether people would have agreed to what is claimed.

The difficulties in getting reasonably good evidence that people would have consented, however, are no reason to reject presumed prior consent arguments generally. To be sure, one may fear that others will overestimate the risks one would have agreed to take. But realizing this, would one demand for a minute that they never try to estimate what one would have agreed to? If others are careful and do not bypass one's actual consent where it is feasible to consult one, and if they do not just indiscriminately refer back without understanding why an earlier time is the important point of reference, attempts to ascertain one's hypothetical will do not disrespect one's autonomy. We should put the matter even more strongly: if others ignore the possibility of presuming one's prior consent, they assault an important dimension of one's freedom amid the imperfect realities of historical social life.

Properly qualified, then, the prior consent model for reconciling clinician loyalty to individual patients with selective denial of their beneficial care rests on sound moral principle. Strong medicine does not always need to wait for people to sign on some dotted line to legitimize a cautious but courageous rationing of care.

NOTES

1. Stone (1985), p. 312.

2. This way of thinking is probably so common among non-strict-constructionist judges and scholars that it never gets spelled out. Dworkin (1986b), pp. 325–26, though he rejects this way of responding to strict constructionism, writes as if it is a major friendly alternative to his own way.

3. Utilitarianism, roughly, holds that acts are right if they maximize the aggregate welfare they create and wrong if they do not.

4. Posner (1980), p. 488.

5. Leonard and Zeckhauser (1986), p. 33. Their exposition of cost-benefit analysis is recent and explicitly addressed to underlying justifications, and Zeckhauser is a long-standing exponent of the method. Note also that the "shadow prices" routinely used in cost-benefit analysis are simply an imagining of the money that consumers would consent to accept if they were selling or buying.

6. Gibson (1985), p. 152.

7. Ackerman (1985), p. 902. Rawls (1971) provides a theory that uses hypothetical persons, not just hypothetical choices.

8. This is also known as the Kaldor-Hicks test.

9. Some economists who urge wealth maximization as a guiding social policy are far from oblivious to this. They claim that either (1) rights claims are dubious in precisely those areas to which wealth maximization is appropriate, as in the case of Factory B, or (2) we may presume that the people affected would have consented to a general wealth-maximization principle. Neither of these defenses of efficiency is likely to succeed. First, even if preexisting rights such as those of the homeowners against Factory A are not at issue, maximizing wealth may not maximize the utility that admittedly has some fundamental moral attraction. Whether wealth is constituted by actual market goods or goods with shadow prices, the standard of monetary value in most economic analysis is a willingness to pay obviously contingent upon income levels. Poor Peter's willingness to pay less than Rich Robert may still leave Peter getting greater utility out of a thing he is paying for than Robert would get. See Dworkin (1980), pp. 196–201. This point is sometimes made (not merely admitted) by defenders of willingness-to-pay models of valuing life; see Menzel (1983), pp. 56–71. Second, not everyone will give prior consent to maximizing wealth in determining what rights people have, even if they are imagined to be taking a distanced view away from the immediate contingency. Poor Peter's and Rich Robert's real chances of cashing in on a significant piece of the admittedly larger economic pie may simply be too unequal to elicit consent to a general policy of wealth maximization from both of them. On this issue, in fact, Posner is quite discriminating. He notes that in some areas of the law wealth maximization may sometimes not result in ex ante compensation, so that there the evidential basis for presuming consent may be missing and wealth maximization not appropriate. See Posner (1980). If, of course, people actually would consent beforehand to a principle of maximizing potential Pareto efficiency, it might indeed have some moral power. The trouble is that such consent is usually simply not there to be presumed. And if it is, it—not potential compensation—is doing all the moral work.

10. This is a simplification of *O'Toole* v. *Greenberg,* 488 N.Y.S. 2d 143 (Court of Appeals of New York, 1985).

11. I am assuming throughout this chapter that agreement was freely made and not coerced. Determining when people's circumstances coerce the choices they make, of course, is an immense and complicated discussion. One of the most sensitive treatments in the context of risk taking regarding health is the discussion of workplace safety by Daniels (1985a), chapter 7, especially pp. 165–76.

12. Coleman and Murphy (1985), p. 270.

13. Coleman realizes this (1980), pp. 534–35. Nino (1983), p. 296, makes essentially the same point about a wider variety of harms, not just crimes.

14. Thomson (1985), pp. 137–38, makes most of these points.

15. An excellent survey of the very sizable literature on this principle is Morelli (1985). Important recent discussions are Simmons (1979), Arneson (1982), and Klosko (1987).

16. Adapted from Nozick (1974), pp. 93–95.

17. Nozick (1974), p. 95, is a bit ambiguous on this last claim. He does not come right out and say that even if she had no better use for her time and would presumably therefore have agreed to contribute, actual consent is still required. He does, though, conclude that "even if the principle [of fairness] could be formulated so that it was no longer open to objection, it would not serve to obviate the need for other persons' *consenting* to cooperate and limit their own activities."

18. "Public goods" are "nonexcludable"—they cannot be provided for some members of a community while being denied to specified others—and depend on the cooperation of large numbers of people. See Klosko (1987), pp. 242–43. "Primary goods" is the well-known label given by Rawls (1971) to goods that everyone is presumed to want regardless of their other individual desires.

19. The traditional notion of "tacit consent" seems closer to acceptance or participation than to the presumed consent I am trying to elucidate. The problem with traditional tacit

consent—for example, consent to state authority allegedly signified by residence—is that it simply does not measure *free* consent. As Dworkin says in dismissing tacit consent (1986b), pp. 192–93, "consent cannot be binding . . . in the way the argument requires, unless it is given more freely, and with more genuine alternate choice." I agree entirely.

20. Virtually this exact example was stated to me by David Eatman (Xavier University of Louisiana). Nozick's book example is similar (1974), p. 95.

21. This is essentially the same reason why hypothetical consent fails in a case cited by Fischer and Ennis (1986), p. 40: "If you consented yesterday to pick me up at the airport today, then you have a moral obligation to do so. But from the fact that you *would have* consented to pick me up at the airport had I asked you yesterday, it does *not* follow that you have any such obligation." We prefer to order our affairs according to the rule that you need not pick me up at the airport unless I arrange that with you. If I do not, I cannot say you are obligated via presumed consent; it is my mistake.

22. Gibson (1985), p. 152.

23. This larger point about the scope of the concept of liberty is from Sen (1983), pp. 18–20.

24. This itself is a presumed consent claim, and therefore the whole argument is in a sense admittedly circular. I do not know how to avoid this, though I am unconvinced that it is a defect.

25. We would want to impose another condition here, but it may not be as obviously relevant to medical rationing cases as the previous one. Actual consent would not be demanded of the citizen in the public-address case if it was thought that she would try to get a free ride by dishonestly exempting herself—a free ride on the vast majority's cooperation by dishonestly refusing consent when she would have to admit that she would contribute her share to the scheme if that was strictly the only way to get the benefits.

26. Paraphrased from Ackerman (1985), p. 903.

27. Dworkin (1986a), pp. 12–13.

28. I have slightly modified case 10 here. In the original case above, the prior consent to restrictive policy was presumed, not actually given.

29. How important? Important enough that if the reasons for using the prior perspective were explained, rational people would agree that it was the right one. See note 24.

3

Consent and the Pricing of Life

People value life in many ways, in many different contexts. *Intrinsically:* We say it is great to be alive. *Relative to other people:* How does the value of my very life compare with yours? The same, probably, but what about an infant's, a child's, or an octogenarian's? *Relative to other things in life:* Do I risk my life to climb this mountain? Should I save on premiums by subscribing to a plan that doesn't cover transplants? How many of its resources should society spend to save me? *As compensation to my survivors if I die:* For how much should I insure my life? What damages should you pay if you wrongfully cause my death?

Responses to these questions express some kind of valuation of life. Some also say something about how the value of life relates to money—they are ways of pricing life, we might say.[1] In modern culture, life innocently gets a kind of monetary value: with a great number of effective but often costly means of preserving life available, we repeatedly trade lifesaving off with other good things, and money mediates the trade-offs.

Such monetary valuation of life seems to be an integral part of rationing. If we put care in short supply, we presumably think that the part we forgo "costs too much"—referring, of course, to the more valuable things we could use the resources for elsewhere.[2] Since life itself is what we would sometimes get if we put more into health care, making medical care scarce really means that we are pricing life. Consent to rationing in particular manifests this clearly: collectively or individually, we impose potentially fatal restrictions on ourselves by putting our marginal money somewhere else.

If we go farther, moreover, and speak of an actual money figure as the value of life—$500,000, let us say—we tie together the whole conceptual package of such resource trading. With such a dollar figure to use as the value of the life that might be saved, then if we spend only the equivalent of that to save what works out to be a life, we can say it is because greater cost would exceed the value produced. Value for money, after all, is what we are after—that even happens to be a common British phrase for costworthy health care. (It is not that independently the value of the thing we would save is less than what we would have to spend to save it, but only that what we have decided to spend to save it is what marks it as having the value we say it has.)

It is hardly strange, then, that economists have often endorsed some way to determine an actual monetary value for people's lives. In recent decades their most popular conceptual model has been *willingness to pay:* the monetary value of life is directly a function of people's willingness to use resources to increase their chances of survival. Suppose one annually demands an extra $500 to perform work that runs an additional 1-in-1,000 risk of dying. Then, according to this model, $500,000 is the monetary value of one's life. Most importantly, this means we need not spend more than $500,000 to save it.[3]

The willingness-to-pay model emerged as a reaction against a "human capital" model that calculated the value of life only in terms of productivity: the present discounted value of one's future earnings.[4] Willingness-to-pay seems infinitely better than that. Its ground-floor use of consent captures not only productivity but the range of life's subjective, intangible value.

This approach may seem eminently plausible conceptually, but that has hardly been enough to gain the model any kind of general moral acceptance. The basic problem is simply that the world in the end is such a different place for a loser than it is for a winner.[5] Suppose one declines to pay the $500 risk-reduction price, taking that 1-in-1,000 risk, and then one dies. In some sense one has consented to what has happened, but did one ever say anything remotely like "less than $500,000 is the value of my *very life,*" the life that is now irretrievably lost? How do we get thrown from an initial trade-off between money and risk to the value of an actual, irreplaceable life?

To be sure, all kinds of impressive defenses of a consent-based, willingness-to-pay model can be mounted:

1. The value of life cannot depend on money, people will say. It is the reverse: without life money is worthless. But could not your willingness to risk death to save money still indicate a real value of life for you when you are alive, even though, if you died, the money would be worth nothing to you?

2. To most people "willingness to pay" mistakenly implies that they would be left to their own financial devices in endeavors such as health care, but the model says nothing of the sort. We can publicly assist those who can-

not afford to pay for health care while using willingness-to-pay values of life to set limits on the medicine then delivered.

3. The willingness-to-pay model need not violate our sense of moral equality by the particular life values it generates. Since the poor are willing to pay less than the rich, the model involves greater monetary values of life for rich people than for poor. But suppose Peter is poor and Robert is rich. The model implies only that the monetary, not overall, value of Peter's life is lower than Robert's, and even then, only in a sense. The value of Peter's life is only lower for Peter, in terms of Peter's own poor person's money, than the value of Robert's life is for him in terms of his money. It would be completely incorrect to think that Peter's is "lower period" or "lower for society" and consequently weigh up Peter's and Robert's monetary life values arithmetically together.

4. There is nothing inconsistent in expressing markedly different money values for one's life in different circumstances. For high-risk situations, for example, Mishan quips that he has yet to meet a colleague "who would honestly agree to accept any sum of money to enter a gamble in which, if at the first toss of a coin it came down heads, he would be summarily executed." At the other end, as the risks one can reduce get very small, willingness to pay drops to zero; if it didn't, one's life-style would be eccentrically cautious indeed.[6] None of this circumstantial variation, however, should be bothersome. It only indicates that life's monetary value is subjective. A consent-based model cannot claim any one value to be correct for all situations, but why should any of its partisans want to claim that in the first place?[7]

Technically all of these defenses seem correct, but a willingness-to-pay model still leaves us uneasy. "His life [now lost] was worth only $500,000"— should we finally actually think things like that? If the prior consent model for restricting health care involves thinking and saying such things, will the model ever be morally acceptable?

This chapter argues that a prior consent approach to rationing lifesaving medicine does not have to make the offensive-sounding claim that the actual value of someone's life is a specific amount of money. First I will make some comparisons by surveying two cultural contexts in which we really do assign monetary values to life: life insurance and legal awards for wrongful death. I will then come back to reviewing the appropriateness of pricing life in contemporary health-care settings. We will learn that the willingness-to-pay approach is not a generally correct method for discerning life's monetary value but that prior consent to risk can still be an appropriate focus for health-care rationing. It does not profane the value of life, and it does not appeal to our darker, irrational side.

A Historical Sidelight: Life Insurance

Moral skepticism about whether life should be perceived as having monetary value is not new. It is interesting to look at an earlier example, the adoption of life insurance. According to Viviana Zelizer:

> Particularly ... during the first half of the 19th century, life insurance was felt to be sacrilegious because its ultimate function was to compensate the loss of a father and a husband with a check to his widow and orphans. Critics objected that this turned man's sacred life into an "article of merchandise." ... Life insurance benefits ... became "dirty money."[8]

Apprehension focused particularly on any commercial pact whose fulfillment depended on death.

Subsequently the marketers of life insurance came to use a very effective strategy: they avoided any talk that smacked of insurance's "profitable investment" and spoke instead only of its moral, altruistic value. Perfectly sensibly, these marketers noted that purchasing life insurance would be making a gift, sacrificing some of one's own consumable income in order to care for dependents. A sermon in the 1880s would later reflect this:

> When men think of their death they are apt to think of it only in connection with their spiritual welfare. ... [But] it is meanly selfish for you to be so absorbed in heaven ... that you forget what is to become of your wife and children after you are dead. ... It is a mean thing for you to go up to heaven while they go into the poorhouse.[9]

Sometimes the language was even more evocative. Life insurance "can alleviate the pangs of the bereaved, cheer the heart of the widow, and dry the orphan's tears," said an 1860 sermon; "it will shed the halo of glory around the memory of him who has been gathered to the bosom of his Father." The U.S. Life Insurance Company's 1850 booklet described it as "the unseen hand of a provident father reaching forth from the grave and still nourishing his offspring."[10]

One can, of course, be cynical about the motivations of the marketers. Because of that, any full sacralization of life insurance will always be impossible.[11] Nevertheless, by the time in the late 1800s when life insurance had taken hold, its marketing could be frank and couched admittedly in economic terms. By then it had already taken on ritual and symbolic functions. "Priceless values were being priced, but the pricing process itself was transformed by its association" with something of fundamental, sacred value.[12] What started out in life insurance as an apparently crass, productivity-focused, "human capital" method of valuing life had been transformed by the now laudable moral purpose it was seen to have.

The parallels to all of this in contemporary health care are striking; only here it is not an adequate productivity substitute but prior consent to risk that gets sacralized. If we derive our limits on what we spend to save life from such consent, have we profaned life? To be sure, if someone greedily encourages us to run those risks to save resources for other things, he or she will be like life insurance beneficiaries who encourage us to take out a wealth of insurance and then smirk with anticipation at our possible demise. So also, if we are sold deviously lean health-care plans by profiteers who cut costs at every corner, surely health care, health insurance, and our lives have been profaned. But just as with life insurance, it does not take much to see things in almost the reverse light.

Containing health-care costs on the basis of prior consent can become noble, moral behavior. We are thereby refusing to let ourselves indulge in an insurance pool's resources merely because we are not immediately paying out of pocket. We are leaving the society or insurance pool with more resources to use on other things—others' lives and health or any dimension of self-respecting quality of life. Even suppose that our motivation for consent to risk is purely selfish—we want more money now with which to pay off bills, to get the car fixed right, to take a vacation. Why not see these as laudably honest assessment of our lives, our finances, and the real sources of our satisfaction?

Thus, far from cheapening respect for life, using consent to risk to see that life has finite monetary value can represent laudable advance. To see life that way may require some marginal cultural shift, but so did our earlier moral acceptance of life insurance. To say that this shift cannot or will not occur is unimaginative indeed. Consent to risk and refusal to pay can indicate an emphasis on quality of life for self and others that reflects a high-minded idealism. This point is admittedly only about possibilities, but that, too, is important.

Wrongful Death Awards

If there is one phenomenon in which society already explicitly puts monetary value on life, it is in awards for wrongful death. The primary function of such awards is to compensate survivors. They may represent more than that; deterrence, efficient prevention, and perhaps retribution are also aims of tort law. But until the mid-nineteenth century, Anglo-American law did not permit any recovery for wrongful death. Even today the highest damage awards are for injuries, not fatalities. Furthermore, in most legal systems the damages for causing the death of someone who has no surviving dependents are next to zero. Thus, as a matter of fact, the primary concern of wrongful death awards has undoubtedly been compensating survivors.[13]

Probably the most bewildering feature of such awards is their wide disparity. Ironically, that may have some mocking logic if a life is irreplaceable and invaluable. On the one hand, if a person cannot be replaced and money cannot possibly make up the real loss, why award anything beyond the tangible financial loss sustained by survivors? Since additional money, no matter how great, cannot make them whole, as lawyers say, do we not profane the value of life by acting as if it can? Yet we might also argue for precisely the opposite conclusion. If we really identify with survivors who have lost a loved one whose life to them is priceless, we can raise awards higher and higher and not worry one bit that we will ever be awarding them too much.

The only way to narrow the disparities in a legal system's actual awards is to assume that lives somehow have a more definite kind of monetary worth for survivors. Actual financial losses caused by death can be calculated (the victim's discounted future earnings, probably, minus his or her own consumption), but these, of course, represent only a portion of the value of a life to survivors.[14] If chaos is going to be taken out of verdicts, we simply have to get some handle on this remaining portion of a life's monetary value. We will have to think in terms of a more basic, comprehensive sense of value for survivors than just productivity.

The broadest of the intangibles for which courts have now increasingly allowed recovery is called *consortium:* guidance, companionship, felicity, sexual relations, and the broad range of benefits each family member would have received from the victim's continued existence.[15] No matter how subjective and intangible these losses are, they are clearly real. This creates an immediately strong case for their inclusion in compensatory awards.[16] But how should we arrive at any specific values for them? When we say, "Here, this is equivalent compensation," what coherent reasoning process could we be reflecting?

Replacements or Equivalent Satisfactions

It might be thought that we are estimating the cost of purchasing truly replaced consortium. However, consortium generally cannot be bought with any price. Perhaps instead what is being estimated is only the cost of obtaining satisfactions of any kind that are equal in amount or degree to those the survivors had in consortium.

But this, too, raises imponderables. What satisfactions of one kind are equivalent to other satisfactions of another kind? Jury members can try to make their own judgments on that point, but in the context of lost consortium with a particular loved one, the whole consideration seems to fall apart.

Willingness to Pay to Reduce Risk

Might prior consent to risk come to the rescue of tort law? Could we ask, for example, what survivors would have been willing to pay beforehand to reduce a given risk of losing their consortium with the victim? To ask this question will probably not quickly cause juries to refuse to cooperate with the very question as we are likely to cause if we ask what money people would take for actually losing a loved one.

Even then, however, such a move would have to be very unsatisfactory for tort law. Tort law aims to make victims or their survivors "whole." Compensation for actual damage is its aim. Just because a survivor would have taken a certain risk of losing the victim in order to retain something else that has determinate monetary value for him or her does not by itself imply that a dollar value computed from that risk acceptance is what he or she has now actually lost as a survivor. In tort law we have to avoid the gap between mere risk on the one hand and the value of actual life lost on the other. Perhaps the closest tort law could get to using prior consent to risk is to throw up its hands. We simply have no other method of arriving at a monetary figure for the value of life lost. Our convictions of fairness insist that survivors must be compensated with something for the clearly real though intangible losses of consortium. So what else can intelligent judges and juries do but refer to survivors' hypothetical prior consent to risk?

Insuring Victims' Lives

We might change the prior consent question as follows: beforehand, what level of compensation for the death of the victim would the survivor have agreed was adequate? Not knowing whether one would end up a survivor to be compensated or the negligent (not criminal) defendant doing the compensating, what would one earlier have agreed to as adequate compensation? To put it another way, what level of insurance would one buy on someone else's life to guarantee one's compensation if that person dies?[17] Admittedly, responses here will not tell us the monetary value of the actual later loss of life. One could always say, "We're supposed to be compensated for actual losses, aren't we? When in saying that I'd risk a loved one's life to save money did I ever imply what the value would be of the *actual* loss I would experience if that person died?" Correct, but one's willingness to insure for only a certain amount does create a moral argument for that level of compensation: one would have agreed to it beforehand.

Interestingly, an argument for keeping wrongful death awards relatively modest now emerges. People tend not to insure fully for the loss of "irreplaceable" commodities. If I make my best estimate of the monetary equivalent of an irreplaceable's value—my spouse, say—I still tend not to insure her for that amount.[18] The likely reasoning is this: "Since money won't be able to replace her completely anyhow, why should I sacrifice a lot else just to get as close as possible to her full value if I lose her? I'll fully insure our house— that will really get us back to square one if it burns down. But when it comes to irreplaceable people, I'll be more stoic." Ironically, then, it is the very irreplaceability of a person's life that has a depressing effect on the insurance value. If hypothetical insurance for compensation is a conceptually correct way to proceed in thinking through awards for intangible losses, then it may bring us back to roughly the same modest figures generated by prior consent to relatively low risks.

Victims' Value to Themselves

Why, though, should wrongful death awards be confined strictly to the victim's value to survivors and not include the more fundamental value to himself or herself? The simple answer is that the victim is dead, so he is not now experiencing any damage, and even if in some sense he were, he is not the one who would be compensated if the value of his life to himself were somehow included in the award. Juries, however, have a tough time swallowing this. Why should a civilly "convicted" defendant get away without paying for the biggest injury of all from her negligence, the one to the victim?

One way tort law could represent the value of the victim's life to himself or herself would be to see it as property transferable to his or her estate. That, though, would raise the legally and morally problematic conception of one's life as property. In the common law generally, not even one's body, much less one's life, is regarded as property. The essential problem is that to own our bodies as property would be to call them things, but we conceptually associate our bodies too intimately with ourselves to find it easy to do that. We are not things, or at least we do not think we should be treated as things. The law has taken this doubt to heart. Courts have subtly negotiated cases about control over bodily materials without calling our bodies property. For example, a plaintiff's blind, unseeing eyeball was temporarily removed for examination for cancer and mistakenly dropped down an open drain in the pathologist's lab. The plaintiff won, but on the basis of his psychological shock upon hearing of the bizarre accident, not because of loss of property.[19] It would then be inconsistent to award compensation for the value of the victim's life to himself or herself, as if the victim's life passed to his or her estate like property.

So where do we come out in all of this? Wrongful death awards cannot be comprised merely of lost future earnings if fair, equivalent compensation is going to be provided to survivors. More intangible personal values of a victim's life also constitute real loss. Yet tort law cannot derive these additional values from risks to the victim's life that survivors might previously have consented to take. Compensation logic looks long and hard for something equivalent to survivors' actual, current losses. The hypothetical insurance that survivors would have taken on a victim's life may get us closer to a morally adequate compensation figure. Since people tend to underinsure for irreplaceable items such as life, the compensation levels from such a conceptual strategy would likely be similar to the modest values derived from prior consent to relatively low risks to life. Tort law cannot easily assess damages for wrongful death by focusing on the value of the victim's life to himself or herself. It could conceivably do that by looking at the person's life as property passed on to his or her estate, but the law has rightfully hesitated to regard bodies as property.

There is a larger lesson here, too. This entire set of puzzles and observations emerges from the dominant purpose of wrongful death awards: fair, equivalent compensation of survivors. For contexts in which the predominant concern is different, such as health care perhaps, our survey of tort law reasoning reveals no precedents for or against the use of prior consent to risk as an indicator of the value of life.

The Different Case of Health-Care Rationing

In health-care rationing prior consent simply does not confront the same problem as in setting wrongful death awards. In health care we do not need to discern a value of actual life already lost. Questions in the health-care context are much more forward-looking.

For example, should $200,000 be spent to add a 40 percent chance of surviving another ten years to an otherwise currently dim prognosis? (A heart transplant might fit facts close to this.) The question here demands no direct evaluation of an actual loss of life. Even in an urgent crisis situation, the issue is still usually one of risks and odds. Furthermore, the money for providing the treatment comes from premiums or taxes that make up a common pool, so the issue becomes in part what policy will allow the pool that the patient has helped create to remain solvent. If as a voter, taxpayer, or subscriber the patient chooses a leaner plan in order to have more money left for other public or private things, his or her consent to subsequently somewhat greater health risks has become a very part of the social and institutional process of providing medical care. Prior consent to risk of life gains no such natural footing in determining wrongful death awards.

Broome's Objection

Not all skepticism about the role of accepting risk in limiting what we spend to save life, though, will be dissolved by such circumstantial facts. One critic, John Broome, claims that in principle only valuations of life made directly in the face of death are correct. They evaluate what actually happens because of a policy; any prior acceptance of risk is only a valuation of the subjective expectations the policy creates. The prior evaluation is useful only to the degree that it approximates its subsequent counterpart. Since most prior valuations of life and death in low-risk contexts yield significantly lower monetary figures than valuations made closer to actual prospective death, the former, Broome claims, are "worthless, and . . . known to be worthless at the time" they are made.[20]

But why, for health-care policy, should Broome be able to claim that a later perspective is correct in principle? Broome only assumes—he does not establish—that in health care, too, valuations of life at times of peril are the proper standard against which prior assessments have to be measured. That temporal perspective may be correct for legal compensation, but why assume that we should always see things that way? To do so automatically in health care simply begs the question of which temporal perspective is most important for making resource decisions. We have already noted[21] the powerful initial reason for thinking that a prior perspective is important in reasonably controlling costs: the time when they subscribe to a plan or vote about public health-care spending is the most effective point at which people can take control over the scarce resources of their lives.

A Verbal Revision

Perhaps, however, there is a correct point to Broome's argument, though it is only verbal: postdeath or in-the-face-of-death judgments must be our point of reference if what we are expressing is properly called the value of *life*. We might doubt that any such verbal requirement was so clear—after all, is not life our focus even in making prior risk decisions? But Broome's view could have a ready answer here: life itself is precisely the first thing people are likely to take for granted. It does require the stark contrast with death before short-sighted, ungrateful human beings can see its real value.

The point is well taken, but Broome's objection has now been reduced to something acceptable to defenders of prior consent: just admit that we made a verbal mistake in calling what we are doing valuing life. We should regard prior consent only as a way of pricing safety, not life.[22] The term *the value of life* was "almost a joke, a bit of gallows humor" inevitably attractive to economists who routinely deal with tragedy-loaded scarcity.[23] Supporters of prior consent should have admitted this all along. That would have enabled us to shed the red herring of offended sensibilities that has dogged consent-to-risk views from the start, without losing anything of substance. A patient previously consented to a lean health plan that now leaves him on his deathbed, and his risk-for-money trade-offs point to a limit of $500,000 per life saved. If we call that an actual "value of his life," are we any better situated to explain why all the stops should not be pulled out now to save his life? We do not have to use any "$500,000 value of life" language at all. The essential point is that the patient consented to something beforehand. The attempted inference—"See, $500,000 is all your life is worth, you said so"—adds nothing morally significant.

Thus, there is simply no need to claim that prior consent to risk generates a monetary value for a specific life. All we need to legitimize prior consent as the proper point of reference is an important reason for binding oneself beforehand for contingencies later. In health care, we have that.

The Remaining Value of Purely Statistical Life

Getting clear on all of this does not prohibit us from ever using prior consent to conceive of a monetary value of life. It still works perfectly well for deriving the value of a statistical life. When we save a truly statistical life, we pay to save just "someone" without ever knowing who in particular that person is. Likewise, if we pass up the chance to save a truly statistical life, we are also ignorant of whose life is finally forgone. Furthermore, even if we do end up knowing who in the end gets fatally exposed, no one has the opportunity to change his or her mind after the earlier, merely statistical choice. Take a cancer, say, which could have been more aggressively screened for; there may just not be any effective choice situation to which anyone can conceptually shift to change ignorance to knowledgeability. The value of life first expressed then sticks all the way through the unfolding process.[24]

Sometimes such statistical lives are the issue in health care—often, say, in prevention—but frequently, as in crisis care, they are not. In either case, prior consent has a crucial role to play in rationing decisions, though we should generally disavow talk of any specific price-of-life figures. Prior consent to risk literally expresses only the value of increased safety, not the value of life itself.

The Rationality of Consent

Consent to risk still faces another severe, directly related challenge. People will usually not "sell" their lives for any amount of money in later high-risk situations, so it is earlier low-risk situations that create enough willingness to risk to get the argument rolling for limits on lifesaving care. But how rational is it for people earlier to agree to part with what they would never agree to part with later for the same likely economic return?

A prior consent model for rationing lifesaving medicine must come clean on this matter. It will have to argue either that there is little that is irrational about these preference variations or that there is nothing wrong with basing rationing policy on irrational preferences. Generally I will take the former approach.

Apparent Irrationalities

Irrational choices under risk are legion. They range from the subtle and complex to the simple gambler's fallacy: if we flip heads ten times in a row, we foolishly think we have more than an even chance of getting tails the next time.[25] Look at part of Allais's paradox in particular. Most people choose (a) a 100 percent probability of gaining $300 over (b) an 80 percent probability of gaining $450, but then they reverse their order of preference and reject (c) a 25 percent probability of gaining $300 for (d) a 20 percent probability of gaining $450.[26] The rational choice in terms of likely dollar payoffs is for d over c, which people do generally make, but it also seems to be for b over a, which they do not. Are they simply inconsistent?[27]

What influences people in choosing a over b is probably an extra margin of perceived value in a gain seen as certain. Because of that we can wonder whether it is really irrational at all to prefer a over b. Psychologists initially raised these cases as threats to rationality, but even Kahneman and Tversky (perhaps the most prominent psychologists in this field) have now left that matter open.[28]

Several interesting theories have been developed to explain how these preference combinations are eminently rational despite their appearance. For example, people may think ahead to different amounts of regret or disappointment that they anticipate they will experience when the results of alternative choices become known.[29] If such analyses work, these various irrational-looking preference combinations paint something far short of the negative picture critics have used to dismiss consent to risk. In a few examples, admittedly, we probably encounter genuine irrationalities,[30] but not as many as we thought.

Knowledge, Imagination, and Attitudes

Where on the spectrum of rationality does consent begin to get moral weight? Everyone could probably agree that consent counts for little when grossly and consistently irrational, but I doubt if we think it must be perfectly rational. To get farther we need to distinguish among degrees and types of rationality.

We might start with a simple breakdown of the components of decisions under uncertainty. One is knowledge of the facts—facts in our rationing context, say, about health care and the health-care economy, including various outcome probabilities. A second element is accurate and vivid imagination of the events that one is risking by a given choice and its alternatives. A third is attitudes toward risk—risk aversion or gambling attraction, for example.

Factual knowledge and imagination are clearly related to notions of rationality and irrationality: an ideally rational decision incorporates full knowledge and imagination. Once we have carefully filtered out any deficiencies in knowledge and imagination, however, attitudes toward risk seem to occupy a largely nonrational status, neither rational nor irrational. For example, when one is risk-averse and prefers option a over b in Allais's problem, one is not irrational if one's preference rests on an extra margin of value one typically experiences from gains that are certain. Or suppose that one is risk-neutral or even a gambler and prefers b over a. One is then also not necessarily irrational. One might just experience an extra measure of value in winning amid uncertainty, an experience that in turn is also not irrational.[31]

Applications

If we use our three basic elements to analyze people's risk-for-money trade-offs, we can make some interesting observations. What, for instance, is involved when people who will not accept millions of dollars to take a 50 percent chance of death will accept a 1-in-1,000 risk to their lives to save $500?[32] Does a failure of knowledge or imagination contribute to the acceptance of risk, or is only an attitude toward risk involved? (Or, in the other direction, does an irrational fear of death lie beneath the refusal of millions of dollars?)

I doubt that there is any general answer. What we can do is try as effectively as possible to impress on people the importance of full knowledge and clear imagination—that is, comprehend the 1-in-1,000 probability, really imagine what eventual loss of one's life would be, understand that in later situations of urgency one might be willing to pay a disproportionately higher price for one's life, realize clearly what one could do with some of the scarce resources one would save by greater willingness to risk, seriously apply what one says one believes about being dead (say, that at worst it is nothingness and certainly not torture), and so on.[33] Having done all that, why still label as irrational the preference of someone who takes more risk proportionate to money saved in an earlier lower-risk situation than he or she is ever willing to take in later imperilment?

Note, though, that we might come to quite a different conclusion about another phenomenon, the way people's implied values of lifesaving often rise sharply as probabilities of harm get extremely small. Suppose one happens to see five dollars to eliminate a risk to one's life as just the basic, minimal amount one will pay if one is going to pay anything, whether the risk one eliminates with it is 1 in 10,000, 1 in 100,000, or 1 in 1,000,000. As those risks descend, the implied limits on the value of saving one's life climb from $50,000 to $500,000 to $5,000,000.[34] What is probably happening here is that one just fails to understand the differences between 1-in-10,000, 1-in-100,000, and 1-in-1,000,000 probabilities. No explanation of how these preferences are rational or nonrational has been developed to displace our suspicion that they simply represent a failure of perception.

No matter how irrational these preferences are, of course, they might still be acceptable if the people affected by consequent allocation decisions have actually held them. Likewise, we may accept people's seemingly irrational actual requests to prolong their dying. Now switch to our current question of whether we would also be justified in following an individual's irrational choice to spend much more to save a life facing a 1-in-100,000 risk than a 1-in-10,000 one? Maybe we would be justified if the people affected had already voiced those irrational preferences, but that is much more problematic if we switch to cases where we have to presume their consent. That is especially the case if we are faced with presuming someone's consent on the basis of empirical data from other people's choices.

Retrieving our three basic elements of consent may throw some light on these matters. If we are going to presume a person's hypothetical agreement, which of these three elements should we allow into our picture of the person whose preferences we are trying to guess? The context is restricted resources, and the individual has already agreed that we should sometimes make allocation decisions on the basis of his or her presumed consent. Would the person want us to read his or her consent as consent with perfect knowledge, with perfect imagination, with no irrational and also no nonrational attitudes toward risk?

I suspect that most people want to be presumed basically but not perfectly knowledgeable. On the other hand, we do want to be seen as having nearly perfect imagination—it more easily fits our common picture of ourselves to be perfectly imaginative and sympathetic than it does to be perfectly knowledgeable. As for attitudes toward risk, I suspect people want them carried into any consent that might be presumed as long as they are nonrational, not irrational. We can hardly pull nonrational preferences out of ourselves without destroying our very personalities.[35]

All of this has interesting consequences. The sharp upturn in implied values of lifesaving as we descend from low to extremely low levels of risk is likely attributable to failures of attention and imagination, so we should not presume those values in the absence of people's actual consent. On the other hand, the reverse variation in implied values of lifesaving between high- and moderately low-risk situations seems to reflect only nonrational attitudes toward risk; they would be perfectly permissible to presume in reading people's hypothetical preferences.

The result seems clear. We may make presumptions about consent on the basis of the generally lower value of lifesaving that people express in moderately low-risk perspectives, perspectives similar to those from which we usually choose insurance or vote for health policy. Rationing gets real bite without pandering to our irrational side.[36]

The Treacherous Use of Empirical Data

How usable is outside empirical evidence about what risks to their lives people would take to save money? Should presumption of prior consent to risk in health care ever take its cue from more general data about willingness to pay? Here, at this very empirical level, prior consent runs into some of its clearest limitations.[37]

In morally counting people's actual consent we should filter out only their most extreme irrationalities, but, as we have seen, in presuming people's consent we should correct for significant knowledge deficiencies and even smaller weaknesses in imagination. And in presumed consent perhaps only rational and nonrational attitudes toward risk should be carried through.

But take, for example, seat-belt studies. An investigator assumes some monetary value for time in buckling up, and then, by examining what risks to their lives people are willing to take to save time, an indirect life-for-money trade-off is calculated.[38] If people know that a fatal accident happens only once in 3.5 million person-trips and a disability only once in 100,000, they may readily choose not to buckle up. They might change their behavior quite dramatically if they were more imaginative and noticed what those odds actually add up to for real people over lifetimes. With 40,000 person-trips in a fifty-year span of driving and riding, one's lifetime likelihood of fatality if one never uses seat belts is nearly one in a hundred and the chance of disability more than one in three.[39]

Labor market studies present an even thornier nest of problems. Suppose a study of high-rise steel construction workers reveals their apparent consent to higher risks for a gain in income amounting to $400,000 for each life lost.[40] This value is probably atypically low, since people who take such jobs are generally not as risk-averse as most.[41] On the other hand, to what segment of the labor market do we look to find more representative data? Some common occupations combine very modest wage levels with surprisingly high risks of death. For example, waiters and waitresses in places where liquor accounts for the majority of revenue run some of the highest occupational risks of death, and bartenders are not far behind. Miners, surprisingly, run somewhat lower risks than bartenders, and roofers take below-average risks; both of these have high wage levels.[42] If many high-risk occupations are associated with relatively low wages, we might even come out thinking that life has a negative monetary value.

This possibility alone should teach us to be wary of simple readings of labor market data for behaviorally revealed preferences. When we look at what workers actually say about the risks they take, we find plentiful comment about inadequate information and frustration at the paucity of other job options.[43] We need accurate measurements of factors such as restricted job mobility and ignorance of risks if we are to make the minimally necessary adjustments in labor market data.

Credible judgments about what price people actually do put on their own lives and safety are thus unusually difficult to come by. Each of these sources of data harbors major difficulties of interpretation. And even if we get any reliable values out of them, we will still not obtain anything like one monetary value for saving life. Consent elicited from one sort of risk perspective is only useful for presuming people's consent in that general type of situation. We can use some allegedly standard monetary value for saving a life only where we have absolutely nothing more specific to go on in estimating people's consent and discerning the sort of risk situation involved. The $750,000 general figure for which Usher pleas, for example, may be a superbly careful extraction from the empirical data that we have, but its usefulness is still extremely limited.[44]

In summary, prior consent to risk will not properly generate any generally usable, specific price of life, but to be relevant to health care it does not need to. It remains a useful conceptual device for deriving allocation policies and blunting health-care providers' moral conflict between overall efficiency and loyalty to individual patients. The way it handles lifesaving decisions is not morally disqualified by the nonrational character of many prior risk preferences, and in a sense it need not even claim to be expressing a monetary value of life itself but only the value of safety. Unlike wrongful death awards to survivors in tort law, it does not need to derive any value of individual life now lost but can approach rationing questions from a more forward-looking perspective. At the point of subscribing to health-care plans people take responsibility for hard choices about their later care, and in voting they give needed direction to legislative and administrative decisions about cost containment.

Furthermore, prior consent is helpful in professionally analyzing certain general allocation questions. For example, it seems to support a very limited priority for remedial over preventive care.[45] Later chapters develop other policy implications—for example, about quality of life in Chapter 5.

Just as more than a century ago life insurance seemed an atrocious affront to the sacredness of life, so also limiting what we now spend to save people with modern health care may seem a morally objectionable, narrow-minded pricing of individual life. But just as life insurance quickly came to be regarded as responsible care for one's survivors, so also consenting beforehand to economic limits on health care can reflect the highest-minded conservation of human resources. It shows no necessary insensitivity toward the things we cherish most.

NOTES

1. More precisely, *price* denotes a selling price to buyers; applied to people's lives, that triggers all sorts of horrors. I use *price* in a more general and colloquial sense, as the numerical monetary value of something even if it is not being sold. On a related difference between *valuing* and *buying,* see Audi (1986), pp. 120–21.

2. There are cases of rationing in which exchangeable resources (money) is not the issue— for example, the rationing of scarce transplantable organs when money cannot increase the supply. I am ignoring these cases here.

3. This is abbreviated. In the case of one's life, one's own willingness to pay to reduce risk is not the whole story. Others are also willing to pay to help one live. Both get added together to generate the monetary value of one's life in the most complete versions of the willingness-to-pay model.

4. For the two seminal pieces that launched the willingness-to-pay model, see Schelling (1968) and Mishan (1971). For the latest in a series of well-known human capital studies, see Rice, Hodgson, and Kopstein (1985). For wide-ranging comparison of the two models and qualified defense of human capital, see Robinson (1986).

5. Dowie (1982), p. 266.

6. This way of putting both extremes is from Mishan (1985), pp. 159–60. Maclean (1986), p. 86, notes that the "pricelessness" of life revealed in the refusal to take any price for sub-

jection to very high risks need not imply that life has infinite value. It may only mean that life is not for sale. See also the section of this chapter on rationality of consent, below.

7. These four points are the essential defense of the model given by Menzel (1983), pp. 24–71. A bigger task would be to defend cost-benefit analysis (CBA) generally. One of the most fundamental questions about CBA is whether differences between offer and asking prices (buying and selling prices) load it toward the status quo. See the exchange between Kennedy (1981) and Markovits (1984).

8. Zelizer (1978), pp. 598, 596. For more details on most of the matters cited here, see Zelizer (1979).

9. T. DeWitt Talmadge, quoted in Zelizer (1978), p. 603.

10. Zelizer (1978), pp. 602, 604.

11. Zelizer (1978), p. 607: "Particularly when it comes to death, to save and to heal is holier than to sell" or to buy. Marketing death will always be seen as somewhat "dirty work."

12. Zelizer (1985), p. 211. Though the quotation is from Zelizer's later book on the pricing of children's lives, the point is the same as the one she makes about life insurance.

13. On the changes in the nineteenth century, see Smedley (1984), pp. 275–80. I owe the argument here to Atiyah (1982), p. 89. I am not denying that standards of negligence might be properly drawn in consideration of efficient prevention but am only saying that once we have decided someone was negligent, we should not set the amount of damages by deterrence or prevention.

14. The financial losses include, of course, the market value of work for which the person would not have been paid but which now has to be done or purchased by survivors (e.g., possibly child care, housework, yard work).

15. See, for example, *Elliott* v. *Willis,* 442 NE 2d (1982, Illinois Supreme Court); and *Sealand Services* v. *Gaudet,* 414 U.S. 573 (1974, U.S. Supreme Court). Consortium is different from grief and bereavement, the direct pain and anxiety caused by death that do not denote the earlier positive value of the victim. In general, see *American Jurisprudence* (1977); Blodgett (1985); and Speiser (1970, 1975). Currently in the United States, total consortium awards of up to $500,000 are not unusual; see Conklin (1984), p. 279.

16. According to legal tradition, only actual losses get compensated, but this does not mean that a compensable loss must itself be financial. Undoubtedly, though, the law thought so for a long time. Zelizer (1985), p. 148, describes legal observers being puzzled when the public in the early 1900s got utterly offended at minuscule awards for blatantly negligent deaths of children: six cents for a New York boy, ten dollars for a three-year-old in Nebraska, and one cent for a twelve-year-old in Missouri. The public, though, might have been right even by the standard of equivalent compensation: while parents endure virtually no financial loss in losing a young child, they usually suffer terrific emotional losses.

17. Hypothetical insurance markets have been used at important points in several well-known philosophical discussions. See, e.g., Dworkin (1981), pp. 297–99, 315–23.

18. Cook and Graham (1977), p. 143, claim this theoretically for insurance of irreplaceable commodities.

19. *Mokry* v. *University of Texas Health Science Center at Dallas,* 529 S.W. 2d 802 (1975). In general, see Dickens (1977), pp. 148–50.

20. Broome (1978), p. 95. See also the reply by Thaler (1982) and the response by Broome (1982).

21. See Chapter 1, third section.

22. One of the founders of the willingness-to-pay model, Mishan (1985), p. 165, now says this explicitly.

23. Usher (1985), p. 168.

24. The statistical/identifiable distinction is notoriously difficult to make precise. I use Usher's definition here (1985), p. 173. Linnerooth (1982), p. 229, notes that in wanting to save an "identified" life we may not want to save a person whose identity we know so much

as to save people, identified or unidentified, whom we know to be in serious peril. For other complications, see Menzel (1983), pp. 159–62.

25. On this and other misperceptions of chance, see Tversky and Kahneman (1982), p. 7.

26. This is very similar to the example used by Tversky and Kahneman (1981), p. 455. The full Allais problem involves another pair of alternatives which puzzle us because of their lower rates of preference reversal from the a/b pair than we find with c/d. For detailed discussion in the context of "disappointment theory," see Loomes and Sugden (1986), pp. 278–80. Other variations of the problem are discussed by Levi (1986), pp. 39–48. For other allegedly irrational phenomena and various sources, see Kahneman and Tversky (1979) and Slovic, Fischhoff, and Lichtenstein (1982). Thaler (1987) is a model summary of categories of systematic error and concludes by pointing to the need for a full descriptive theory. For a more popular sort of summary, see *QQ* (1988).

27. Sugden (1985b) has correctly argued that the traditional transitivity standard for consistency of preferences is not necessary to rationality. The inconsistency involved in the example above, though, is of a different sort.

28. Kahneman and Tversky (1982), p. 173 (concluding paragraph). Levi (1986), p. 47, claims that the Allais and Ellsberg problems gained great initial interest not so much because respondents departed from strict maximize-statistically-expected-utility principles but because their responses also seemed to have something very right and rational about them.

29. On "regret theory," see Bell (1982) and Loomes and Sugden (1982). On "disappointment theory," see Loomes and Sugden (1986). On both, see Loomes (1986).

30. For example, people who are willing to drive across town to save five dollars on a ten-dollar calculator are often unwilling to drive as far to save the same five dollars (or even ten dollars) on a hundred-dollar jacket. See Tversky and Kahneman (1981) and Kahneman and Tversky (1982).

31. Sugden (1985b), p. 174, makes the same point about the disappointment/elation and regret/rejoicing that people experience in the results of risk decisions.

32. There are really two things going on here. Implied values of saving a life vary both with the level of risk we are trying to reduce and the size of the reduction available. See Jones-Lee (1974); Weinstein, Shepard, and Pliskin (1975); and Linnerooth (1982), pp. 232, 236.

33. Critics tend to forget the last two irrational oversights. I am not being fanciful in raising them. How often do people think hard about what a fifty-dollar saving in their monthly health insurance premiums could actually do in other uses? Many are content to let it ride as an "invisible" deduction or fringe benefit.

34. Blomquist (1982), p. 36; and Mishan (1985), pp. 161–62; among others.

35. There is admittedly a fundamental philosophical problem here. Can the ultimate foundation of our choices be simply nonrational desires? See Hollis (1983), especially pp. 254–57, for discerning puzzlement over the need of autonomous personalities for some non-arbitrary perspective with which to anchor themselves.

36. Throughout this section I have benefited from Audi (1986), pp. 117–23.

37. The first question to decide in gathering any empirical data will not be pursued here: whether to look to people's actual behavior or their stated preferences. This is not merely a controversy among empirical investigators about whether questionnaires or behavior will provide the most accurate data. We first have to decide what it is we are trying to measure. But that more basic query is moral and philosophical: is the morally relevant consent manifested in behavior, or is it a consent of reflective statement?

38. See also Ghosh, Lees, and Seal (1975), inferring the value of lifesaving from people's choice of highway travel speed.

39. Slovic, Fischhoff, and Lichtenstein (1982), p. 480.

40. The revision of Thaler and Rosen (1976) by Bailey (1980), adjusted to 1985 dollars.

41. Viscusi (1978).

42. For surprising comparisons and an interesting explanatory account, see Graham and Shakow (1981). See also Brown (1980) and Graham, Shakow, and Cyr (1983).

43. Brown and Nelkin (1984). For an excellent summary of and extrapolation from many other interesting details in Brown and Nelkin, see Anderson (1988), pp. 58–63. For constructive analysis of adequacy of information, see Viscusi (1983), pp. 59–75. On workers' rights to know and employers' duties to reveal, see McGarity (1984). The entire labor market data problem is complicated by the relative invisibility of safety and the visibility of envy-creating wages; see Frank (1982).

44. Usher (1985), p. 191.

45. For the full argument and qualifications, see Menzel (1983), pp. 169–74.

4

The Costs of Lifesaving: What If Smoking Saves Money?

What Counts as a Cost of Life?

When we wonder whether the cost of lifesaving measures is worth paying, we typically think of their nominal, direct cost. We also work readily with net cost, discounting direct cost by what we save in the often sizable medical expenditures we avoid.

There are, in fact, many other monetary costs of saving life. Some of them are the ordinary costs of living in the years of life we add—the sorts of things we figure in monthly budgets, for example. These hardly cross our mind when we wonder whether a particular segment of health care costs too much. "Death is a very good way to cut down on expenses," says Woody Allen,[1] but we laugh precisely because we do not think for a minute that the savings he refers to are any reason to welcome death.

Generally, economic analysis tends to widen our commonsense view of medical costs. First it conceptualizes cost as opportunity cost, the best alternative use we forgo by using our resources in one way rather than another. (Theoretically it is already opportunity cost that is reflected in the market cost of goods and services. We have to offer the money for them that we do in order to entice the resources they require away from next-best uses.) In the case of medical care, those alternative uses may have entirely non-health-related purposes. Furthermore, in formalizing the value of life, economic analysis has sometimes counted a person's earnings as one of the ordinary monetary benefits of being alive.[2] That is a big foot in the door: if a forgone benefit of life—future earnings—counts as a kind of opportunity cost of death, why don't the equally obvious ordinary costs of living that are saved when a person dies count as opportunity benefits of death?

Once we think about it, in fact, counting absolutely all costs and benefits, no matter how ordinary or distant they might be, has such a strong theoretical attraction that the only thing that keeps us cautious is the need to avoid hidden double-counting. But though we might want to agree quickly to a completely comprehensive counting policy, we should think through its implications carefully. They can be disturbing.

For any lifesaving program or procedure, with a comprehensive cost-counting approach, we would not just take its nominal price and discount that by what is saved in avoiding care otherwise required. We would also add in all the costs that people incur in living longer because of the program in question. Two such costs will often be especially large: additional pension payouts and all the later, unrelated health-care expenses they will run up in the course of their longer lives.

Antismoking programs provide a particularly striking illustration of what happens. Smoking is probably the single most preventable health hazard in the United States, responsible for one in every four deaths,[3] yet, because the most serious smoking diseases tend to occur near the end of people's earning years, lost work time from illness and lost earnings from premature death are not as high as we might expect. Costs of smoking then fall into the range where they can even be outweighed by the additional health-care expenses and pension payouts run up in the longer lives of people who are persuaded to quit smoking or never to smoke.

Without making any sort of empirical study, we can gain some sense of the costs of smoking in actual numbers from the literature. It is not clear that smoking finally creates any net economic cost at all. First, the common claim that smoking increases medical costs is probably mistaken if it refers to the long-term, overall costs of smokers' as compared to nonsmokers' care. In one well-known study, expected lifetime medical expenditures for typical smokers age thirty-five turned out to be 6 percent less than those for similar nonsmokers.[4] Admittedly, in terms of annual per capita costs, smokers probably do run up greater costs, and the trivial claim that in a given year of life a smoker is likely to incur higher expenses than a nonsmoker is undoubtedly true. However, nonsmokers probably pay a lower portion of their total lifetime health-care costs than smokers do, even after accounting for smokers' higher lifetime contributions in taxes and premiums.[5]

Furthermore, the highest single cost of most smoking-reduction programs may be additional pension payouts decades later.[6] Combined with later health-care costs these mean that smokers are probably not imposing any net costs on others.[7] These two items turn almost any effective antismoking measure from a hoped-for money-saving device for government back into what is still for it a costly program. This is probably most shocking when we realize that a "smokers, pay your share" argument for special tobacco taxes might get turned around 180 degrees: if smokers pay for more than their own lifetime health-care expenditures and pension benefits and it is nonsmokers who really run up higher costs, maybe nonsmokers ought to compensate smokers.

The larger question here is not at all smoking-specific. Smoking only happens to be an interesting, current example which has received great political and social attention, and it illustrates the underlying issue well because of its particular age-mortality impact. Smoking diseases typically kill people early but not too early, before longer years of pension payouts and health-care expenses of general old age but near the end of people's earning years.[8] In addition to smoking there are plenty of diseases and procedures for which what to count as a cost also makes a major difference. Unrelated later health-care expenses turn the screening of low-income elderly women for cervical cancer from a program that certainly should be adopted because it actually saves society money into only a marginal bargain costing roughly $8,000 per year of life saved.[9] A more significant example given the increasing importance of long-term nursing-home care may be the routine vaccination of elderly residents for influenza. A noted economic analysis of influenza immunization for the U.S. Medicare population showed direct costs of only $13 per year of healthy life saved.[10] At that price, how could any sane Medicare administration fail to cover routine use of flu vaccine? Even including the costs of later unrelated health care (but not long-term nursing-home expenses) for patients whose lives the immunization prolongs increases cost to only $800 per year of healthy life—still an incredible bargain. But the inclusion of longer years of social security payouts and nursing-home bills may bring costs to a level where the case for not covering vaccination becomes plausible.[11] Perhaps it is, in fact, the worry about additional years of medical expenses, nursing-home bills, and social security benefits that actually explains why the Medicare administration and Congress have been so reticent to cover routine vaccination.

The aim in this chapter is to sort out this general matter of whether and when to count later health-care expenses and pension payouts as costs of saving life. Because of its important place in the larger economic picture, we will also have to examine a third element: a related benefit of living longer—future earnings.[12] In this discussion antismoking measures will be the dominant practical backdrop until a final section shifts to flu vaccine for nursing-home residents.

Concerns throughout can be divided into two different questions, one conceptual and one moral. The conceptual question is whether a given item—say, pension payments—really is a cost. The moral question already assumes that the item in question is a real cost but still asks whether we ought to count it in the economic assessments that help us prioritize health-care investments.

We will also have to distinguish another pair of questions, each appropriate for quite different policy contexts: what counts as·an *external cost* (a cost to others—other people than the patient or the smoker, for example), and what counts as a *cost overall* (a cost to society, considering everyone). Though because of fair taxation concerns, the former, external cost question will tend to predominate in the discussion of smoking, the other cost-to-everyone question remains important, too. And in the section on nursing homes, the cost-to-everyone question will predominate. Any conclusions will be explicitly attached to one or both of these two different cost questions.[13]

The Quick Solution for Smoking Costs

Would it not be easiest just to accept the principle of counting all the different sorts of costs previously mentioned and then simply shift the case for anti-smoking measures to the positive value of the life they save? Suppose it eventually cost $100 billion to reduce the incidence of smoking by 40 percent, adding an average year of healthy life for each of 20 million people.[14] That is $5,000 per year of healthy life saved, a reasonably good bargain as lifesaving measures go. Let's just count all the program's costs and attend to what we usually do in health policy discussions: is the amount of life saved worth that expense?[15]

This looks like a valid, quick solution to the problem of how to count costs of anti-smoking programs. It is honest, for one thing: if something is a cost, count it. But it does not resolve all of the questions about cost counting.

First, the real cost status of pension payouts will still remain an issue. Economists have traditionally not regarded them as a true cost. They are a cost to government and premium payers, of course, but are they a cost to society, to everyone affected? Are they not there only a transfer, not the using up of some resource[16] but only its shift from one person's control to another's? Contrary to much habit in economics, however, the matter may not be that simple. If people live longer and draw more social security benefits, it seems obvious that they use more resources without in any sense replacing them. We still have an interesting conceptual issue to settle.

Second, the political and moral case for some smoking-reduction measures requires the assumption that smokers do not pay their fair share of costs—that they create a net cost for others. U.S. Surgeon General C. Everett Koop's argument for achieving a tobacco-free society by the year 2000, for example, appeals to eliminating not only massive death, suffering, and disability but "an economic burden we can no longer bear."[17] Health education campaigns and prohibitions on advertising and distribution to children[18] can be based on protecting consumer liberty, but adult advertising restraints may need something such as Koop's cost-to-others assumption, and higher tobacco taxes certainly do.

Adult advertising restraints are usually defended by saying that smokers have irrational addictions not protected under the banner of liberty, but the contrary case for "rational addiction" at least deserves consideration. Maybe *addiction* simply indicates smokers' enhanced pleasures from tobacco, their greater subjective withdrawal costs, and their higher personal discount rates.[19] If smokers who continue to smoke are thus not irrational, advertising restraints may need to fall back on balancing the otherwise unfairly uncountered appeals of powerful tobacco companies,[20] on the impossibility of restricting advertising that directly affects children and adolescents without restricting advertising to everyone, or on the extra costs that smoking allegedly imposes on others. The first two of these fallback reasons would seem to justify only counteradvertising or selective restrictions, not the total ban on television advertising currently in place in Britain and advocated in the United States by Koop. Thus, the final case for advertising restrictions may still involve some claim about the net costliness of smoking to others.

But in any case, the justification of often-proposed greater taxation of tobacco products rests more clearly on the alleged costliness of smoking to others. The theoretically persuasive argument for special excise taxes is that people ought to pay their fair share.[21] Assuming that starting or continuing to smoke are ultimately free choices,[22] fair share means the *full* share of marginal net costs. It is thus objectionable if smokers shift onto others the economic cost they create, a situation that special taxes are needed to correct.[23]

Advocates of tobacco taxes may think they can avoid pay-your-fair-share arguments by relying only on efficiency considerations, but they cannot. The standard efficiency justification for excise taxes also starts off with claims about long-run external costs. When consuming a good creates costs for others, buyers will purchase more than is really efficient, basing their decision as they do only on their private, not the total, cost. A tax is thus needed to raise the consumer's private cost closer to total cost and encourage consumption at a more efficient level.

Because of the importance of the external costs of smoking in both the fair share and efficiency arguments, then, tobacco tax policy simply must deal with how to compute these costs. Specifically, should the cost of a nonsmoker's health care and pensions in added years of life be deducted from the more direct costs that a smoker creates for others? We might try to avoid this question by focusing just on social costs (costs to everyone), generously counting all costs and then nonetheless justifying antismoking measures by the value of life they save. But even if the value of that life outweighs the most inclusively calculated costs, any nonpaternalistic argument for particular measures such as special tobacco taxes still requires the assumption that smoking creates net costs to others.

Right here, though, someone is likely to try a reductio ad absurdum objection to pursuing this external costs discussion. It may seem right to see the case for tobacco taxes as strictly depending on the assumption that smoking is finally costly to others. But would we not then be saying that if *not* smoking turns out to be more costly behavior for others than smoking, a government would be justified in adopting reverse measures to make nonsmokers pay *their* way? Might that not include subsidies *for* tobacco or even government-sponsored cigarette advertising?[24] Do such outlandish possibilities not constitute a reductio ad absurdum objection to this entire discussion of external costs in economic assessments of lifesaving programs?

Fortunately, a direct and essentially simple response can ward off this objection. There is an important moral difference between two government behaviors:

1. A government fails to subsidize or advertise a product, though its use is cheaper to others than nonuse.
2. Though its use is cheaper to others than nonuse, a government still taxes a product or prohibits its advertising.

The fair share objection is persuasive against the second sort of government behavior. Why should others tax one's use of a product if one's use is already cheaper for them than nonuse? In the first case, by contrast, the fair share objection is suspicious. How can people correctly accuse one of causing them an unfair disadvantage just because one voluntarily does *not* use something? For one thing, there are thousands of things people do not use that might reduce others' costs if they did.

So we can proceed. We wonder what a real cost is, and the external costs justification of certain antismoking measures demands that we sort out more carefully just what should be counted in the cost of smoking to others. I will take up later health-care expenditures, future earnings, and pension payouts, in that order.

Later Health-Care Expenditures

Economist Louise Russell has argued against counting later health-care expenses. If the question is what a preventive program means for future medical expenditures, they should be counted. But if the purpose of the analysis is . . . to determine whether the program is a *good investment,* only the costs of the preventive program [itself] should be counted. Added years of life involve added expenditures for food, clothes, and housing as well as medical care. None of these is relevant. . . . Future medical expenses are one of the indirect consequences of the health gains from a program. . . . They are not an addition to health effects.[25]

Russell is making two different arguments here.

Indirect Consequences versus Health Effects

Looking at issues from an economist's wider "social point of view," we want to assess the place of deliberate health programs in the whole economy. Russell does not explain why even from that perspective the distinction between "health effect" and "indirect consequence" should matter, but perhaps her view is explained by a hidden moral assumption. Her distinction may be an instance of the more general difference between intended and merely foreknown effects, the well-known doctrine of double effect: though one *foresees* the later unrelated health-care expenses of another person's added life when one encourages that person to quit smoking, one surely does not *intend* to create them. One intends them neither as an end nor as a means to what one aims at (the other's longer life). They are only side effects.

But if this is Russell's argument, it doesn't help her final case much. The moral significance of the difference between intended and merely foreknown effects is itself notoriously debatable.[26]

The Parallel with Food and Clothing

If someone proposed to count future food and clothing costs in deciding whether to save a life, would one's reaction not be precisely what Russell needs? ("You can't count those, they're just part of what anybody needs to live!")

This reply does not deny that food and clothing are actual costs. It only makes a moral claim about them. When people continue to live, they should not in any way be held accountable for using up financial resources for the bare essentials of life, because anyone who lives has a right to those. Suppose one lives longer. Thus alive, one certainly cannot be expected to reduce or eliminate the consumption of bare essentials. But later medical care is just as much a necessity as food or clothing, so if one should not be charged with using up resources in living longer to eat and be clothed, one should never have to justify one's use of resources in later medical expenses. That holds regardless of whether the focus is total costs to everyone or just external costs.

This argument is deeply embedded in our common reactions to this cost-counting issue, but it is beset with problems. Granted, minimal food, clothing, shelter, and health care are one's rights in the time during which one is already assumed to be living. But why, just because that is true, must we ignore their costs when the matter at issue is explicitly the extension of one's life? Admittedly, food is a necessity to which people have rights partly or even largely because it is essential to their living longer, not merely to enjoying the life they have already. Still, is there not a difference between rights to things when being alive is an assumed background condition and rights to those things when extension of life is the issue? If we had a distinct shortage of food, for example, would we not see to it first that people who were going to live a considerable time anyhow got sufficient food to avoid lingering malnutrition? Would we not think it crucial to count food in figuring the cost of the years of life added by particular lifesaving measures?

So Russell's parallel-with-food-and-clothing argument, while cogent, is limited. The more that basic necessities themselves are seen to be scarce, the weaker the argument gets. If there are sufficient resources to provide everyone with minimal food and clothing, even those who might live longer, we should not consider the cost of such essentials. On the other hand, if we regard such essentials as themselves scarce, we are hardly attracted to the argument at all.

We might also see conscious decisions to adopt lifesaving programs as significantly different from the natural continuance of people's lives. The greater the difference we see between just continuing to live and deliberately adopting lifesaving programs, the weaker Russell's food-and-clothing argument gets.

Furthermore, we might not see the later health care whose expense is at issue to be a clear necessity. The argument demands that later medical care be regarded as essential or strictly minimally decent—that is, as care to which people have virtually as strong a right as they have to food. In the current day, when many people are giving various categories of care low enough priority to regard them no longer as necessities, no wonder we are attracted to counting the health-care expenses of added years of life.

How does the food-and-clothing objection finally stack up? It applies to both total cost and external cost contexts, but in either case our philosophical and cultural perceptions weaken its force. It falters as our perception of health care as a common essential in added years of life diminishes, as we view health-care resources themselves as scarce, and as we see deliberate life extension to be different from life's natural continuance. We are probably now located somewhere near the middle of this philosophical cultural landscape. The objection is bothersome but not persuasive.

Counting Later Health-Care Expenses Later

Beyond these two versions of Russell's argument, there is another possible objection to counting later health-care expenses. Whether the context is overall costs in society or costs to others, is not later the proper time to count them? Since people will then be deciding whether the human benefit of that care is or is not worth what it costs, we should face up to its economic justification *then.*

This may seem correct, but consequently not including these later statistically predictable medical expenses in assessing current lifesaving programs would require unusual and incredibly cumbersome cost-counting procedures. We would have to exclude from the benefit side of our current assessment all the life and health benefits of the later care, counting now only the benefits achieved *between* now and then. In the world of statistical estimates of what life a particular program buys, how could we separate those two things? It would seem much more sensible just to assume that any later health care will buy sufficient benefits to be worth its cost then and consequently count now both the costs and the benefits of that later care.

Finally, should we count later health-care expenditures as a cost of lifesaving? Generally, probably yes. The first and third arguments above provide little reason for excluding them. The second, the parallel with necessities such as food and clothing, is more promising, but it is limited by various cultural and philosophical contingencies. These conclusions hold for both total and external costs.

Future Earnings

Later health-care expenses counted as a cost of lifesaving could be at least partly canceled out by extra future earnings[27] counted as a benefit. Thus, with some lifesaving programs it may make little difference whether we count both or neither. What would more likely make a big difference would be to count one but not the other—later health-care expenses as a cost, say, but not future earnings as a benefit. In the previous section I generally argued for counting later health-care expenses. What about future earnings as a benefit?

There is a strong theoretical reason for counting one once we count the other. If the first reason for counting later medical costs is simply that they are a real consumption cost, we should count future earnings as a benefit; they represent a real addition of goods and services.

This may appear to settle the matter, but there is the nasty problem of unwitted double-counting. This is Russell's objection. Future earnings are only one of the consequences of the health effects of a program. Good health and longer life are valuable partly because they allow people to remain productive workers longer. There are ... other reasons as well. ... All of these are implicit in the estimates of health effects. Estimates of earnings help to describe the consequences of better health in greater detail, but they are not an addition to health effects. To include them as a separate item is to count some of the effects twice—once as a gain in health and again as a saving to be subtracted from program costs.[28]

Whether future earnings have already been counted, however, depends on how we understand "health effects." We might not try at all to convert their value to monetary form but just continue to see them in their health benefit units—years of healthy life, let us say.[29] An economic assessment of health care then comes out telling us a procedure's cost and the years of life it will produce; we compare that with the cost/health-benefit ratios of other procedures and make some decisions, without ever converting the years of extra life into economic currency. It seems we have *not* already considered future earnings in "health effects."

Russell would still have a valid point, though, if we were putting an explicit money value on the years of life themselves. Suppose that in evaluating the extra life in monetary terms we used some version of the willingness-to-pay model.[30] People undoubtedly already account for some of their future earnings when they are or are not willing to pay to reduce risk, but it is not easy to generalize how much. Other more intrinsic values of life may drive most of their conscious preferences here, but anticipated earnings undoubtedly influence the monetary range within which their preferences fall. For the part of future earnings that people use for consumption, Russell seems correct in charging double-counting.[31] People have already reflected much of this in the "enjoyment of life" dimension naturally captured by willingness to pay.[32]

But I suspect that now we have unnecessarily complicated the process we actually go through in the use of cost assessments of health care. If the value of life is regarded as one of the components in the economic calculation itself, then, yes, most future earnings may already be included in the dollar value assigned to life. But the process is more likely as follows: we first obtain an estimate of a lifesaving program's comprehensive, long-run, net monetary costs ("economic" costs in colloquial language), so we can then decide whether the ostensibly nonmonetary value that paying those costs gets us is worth them. In such a procedure, should we not include future earnings in calculating the net economic consequences that set the stage for our final, essentially noneconomic evaluation?[33] I do not see how this would involve us in double-counting.

If we are clear on all this and have appropriately guarded against double-counting, we should count future earnings in the basic net cost assessment.

Lost Surplus Earnings: A Real External Cost

Another consideration weighs in favor of counting the part of lost future earnings beyond self-consumption: a person's surplus earnings, we might call it.[34] Losing those earnings is an external cost of premature death, and recouping them is a benefit of lifesaving. It would be self-defeating for others concerned about their costs not to count these earnings, since they usually gravitate eventually back to them. If surplus earnings are not going to be counted again in a final value-of-life judgment, then not to count them earlier in overt cost calculations could lead people to reject programs that seem to cost them too much but do not really do so. They would be shooting themselves in the foot, trying to make decisions about others' lives on the basis of costs to themselves yet ignoring some of the real benefits that eventually come their way. So in external cost contexts, surplus future earnings should be counted.

Income Discrimination

One dominant challenge remains. Future earnings, it will be argued, over-represent people with higher incomes and underrepresent those with lower incomes. This may or may not be a telling argument, and I will not critically pursue it to any general conclusion. Here I will only note what we should be aware of in a context that focuses on external costs.

What does the choice of counting or not counting surplus future earnings really amount to? If we do not count them, we run the danger of passing over some health-care programs because of perceived high cost to us which is actually much lower. Excluding surplus future earnings would effectively lead us to pay less (net) in available social resources to save a high earner's life than we pay to save the life of a low earner.[35] The point is not that we should automatically include surplus future earnings and disregard their obnoxious-looking effect of giving an advantage to higher-income groups. We should, however, realize that their exclusion would really amount to a willingness of people to pay higher long-run net costs to save low earners than high earners.

As an external cost, surplus future earnings should be counted; that is not double-counting. Excluding them would have to involve a much wider-ranging philosophical argument that future earnings unfairly advantage high earners. As for total costs, we should be wary of double-counting if we include future earnings, but even here the usual process of making health policy decisions after first receiving a comprehensive estimate of net economic cost allows us to include all earnings without confusion in that preliminary calculation.

Pensions

For smoking, at least, counting later pension payouts probably influences the bottom line on costs more than anything else. Here again, essentially two sorts of objections arise: moral objections and conceptual ones (are pension payouts really economic costs at all?). I will first examine the conceptual objection that pension payouts are costless transfer payments. Then I will take up more briefly two moral objections.

Transfer Payments

A virtually standard assumption among economists is that as transfer payments, pension benefits are not overall costs from the social point of view. Though someone through taxes or premiums pays them to someone else, society—everyone, all of us together—loses nothing.[36] When people die, they have lost a pension benefit, but the rest of us have saved a roughly equal expense. Either way, this contrasts with consumption, whereby real uses of goods and services are involved.[37]

This view is correct if we are comparing two courses of events among the same population. Either one transfers to another and the other is clearly there to gain as much in value as one would have, or one keeps what one has and the other gets along without, though there, too, the other is still around. I do not want to challenge this traditional explanation of why pensions are virtually costless for the typical set of circumstances it assumes. But I do want to challenge this view for other settings.

Things look different when we compare courses of events in which the number of people has changed. That is exactly what happens in lifesaving programs. In them we are comparing (a) a course of events in which one is alive to receive a payment from others, with (b) a course in which the others save that expense, but not because one is doing without—one is just not around at all.

Compared to the second, is the first a cost? To the others, of course, it is (so it is clearly an external cost), but that is not our concern here. Is it a cost from the social point of view? There is an obvious sense in which it is neutralized by being a benefit to one, yet only a sense. In the second course of events, in which one dies, there are fewer people among whom the goods and services will be spread. Someone somewhere down the economic line is going to have more there than in the first situation, without anyone in the second getting less. In this respect, b is a gain compared to a, and a is a cost compared to b.

The easiest way to describe this respect is probably to say that per capita net income is lower in a. This does not refer to one's per capita income, or another's, but to per capita income generally. The frame of reference is completely societywide. So in one larger societal sense, pensions are real costs. Of course, whether it is per capita income or aggregate income that ought to be considered is then itself the important and open question. Perhaps most economists focus more on aggregate than on per capita benefit because of the impersonal sense of value with which they typically work. I suspect that most people, though, lean more toward a per capita perspective.[38]

There are ways to escape this conclusion that pension benefits are per capita real costs, but they do not readily hold for smoking-reduction programs. One is an "overlapping generations" view of pension schemes. Suppose someone develops a cure for cancer that lengthens one's life, and one absorbs more pension benefits. Tax or premium payers have to do with less for their own current consumption, but they, too, will see themselves as likely to share in that life-extending benefit—everyone identifies with the risk of getting cancer. Because the expense of living longer can always be passed on to a new generation, which in turn can pass it on to another, everyone recoups what is initially lost. The first generation in on this development, of course, is better off yet, but no one ever loses.[39]

The problem with applying this view to antismoking programs, however, is that most people do not benefit from them enough to make up for their higher social security taxes. Literally, of course, a cancer cure does not benefit most people either (most people do not get cancer). But most people do easily see themselves as potential cancer victims (non–lung cancer, that is). Generally, I doubt if people identify with each other nearly as much on the smoking issue. If one person quits smoking, another is more likely to mind the first person's higher pension benefits than he or she would if a cure was found for the cancer. "I, too, might have had cancer" comes more readily to our lips than "I, too, might have smoked and then quit." We do not identify with each other enough on smoking to use the overlapping generations model and see everyone as a winner.

There is another way to save the costless transfer payment view, but it, too, is problematic. Suppose the missing person in the second course of events above would have injected additional goods and services into the first course had she lived: some distinctive labor in old age—cheering up children, for example, or teaching others the subtle lessons of gracious appreciation. She pulls out more pension benefits in her added years of life, but creates fully compensating, equivalent goods.

But *equivalent* goods is a tall order. By hypothesis these goods are not created through paid economic productivity, nor are they hidden in the value of life already counted for added years. They have to reside in some other kind of value from the pensioner's longer life. Without them the pension payouts of added years of life still emerge as real costs to others.

Thus, from one sort of larger social point of view—aggregate income—additional pension benefits aren't real costs. But from another, equally societywide perspective—per capita income—they are real costs. And in any case they are real costs to others.

The next two objections to counting additional pension payouts can probably best be understood against the background of this conclusion. They argue against counting additional pension payouts even if we have concluded that they are real costs and costs to others is our concern.

We've Paid for Them

The paradigm here is an annuity pension, where one pays in roughly as much as one is statistically likely to draw out. The fund will probably require one to pay higher premiums the longer one is expected to live. If one paid in what the fund asked, and if the fund chose not to charge more when it could have, then one would seem to have as much right to additional years of payouts as one does to earlier ones. If one lives longer as a nonsmoker, only in a weak sense are one's higher pension benefits external costs that are passed on to others—one defrayed them already in the pension one purchased. In any case, one is entitled to them. Why, therefore, should a smoking reduction program that benefits one be required to carry these costs into its policy debate?

This argument is familiar and its limitation clear: it works to exclude additional pension payouts from our cost counting only when they are part of annuity pensions. Neither British old-age pensions nor American social security pensions are. They admittedly have some collective annuity dimension: since people paid into the system all those years, they have a right to get out something close to what was projected for them. But that projection is not based straightforwardly on what any particular person paid in, so people can hardly expect others to ignore any higher payouts they run up.

Pensions as Rights

The argument here is similar to the parallel-with-food-and-clothing objection to counting later health-care expenses. If society sets up a nonannuity pension scheme because it thinks people have a right to be assured that base of support regardless of their private arrangements, why should it count pension costs against one when one lives longer and draws out what one has a right to draw out?

Again, however, we return to the difference encountered earlier in the food-and-clothing objection to later health-care expenditures. One may have a right to a pension benefit for the time when one is alive, but that hardly commits us to saying that one has a right to have one's life *extended* without regard to the impact one has on others by drawing the benefit. We may not see much of a difference between these two sorts of rights in the case of food, clothing, and really basic medical care. Insofar as pensions have been set up in order to provide for such equally basic needs as these, they will carry with them the force of the parallel with food and clothing. The parallel will deteriorate, however, to the degree that a pension program's benefits are not really needed by its recipients. Currently in the United States, in fact, that consideration is very much at issue; social security benefits are often no longer regarded as going primarily to those in need.[40]

Should the public pension benefits in longer years of life be counted as a cost of lifesaving programs? They are costless transfer payments from an aggregate income perspective, but from an equally societal, per capita perspective they are real costs. They are virtually always real costs to others. To say of public pension benefits that we have paid for them is no objection to their being counted in either general or external cost contexts. For either sort of context, to say that pensions are rights still leaves open the question of how basic a necessity they are for most of their recipients; people might have rights to them but not in so strong a sense that their cost ought to be excluded when the policy question is extending life.

The Limits of Health Promotion

I have pressed two sorts of queries. First, are added years' health-care expenditures and pension benefits real costs, future earnings real benefits?

1. Later health-care expenses are real costs.
2. Future earnings have sometimes already been counted implicitly in economic assessment. When lifesaving preserves them, however, that is a real benefit that still needs explicit counting in the more typical process of first estimating net monetary cost before judging whether a program's less economic benefits are worth that cost. In any case, surplus earnings beyond self-consumption need to be counted in calculating net external costs.

3. Additional pension payouts are not real parts of the aggregate social cost of lifesaving, but they are real per capita costs. Generally they are also a real cost to others.

So at least in some important contexts all three of these are real costs and benefits. Second, however, ought we as a matter of morally defensible social policy to count them? This is considerably more complex.

4. Later health-care expenditures are rather indirect consequences of lifesaving, but in either total or external costs this would argue against counting them only if we generally thought the distinction between intended and merely foreknown results was morally correct.
5. Pensions may be rights, but to say that they therefore ought not to be counted is persuasive only on a very strong assumption about the kind of rights they are.
6. The arguments that have a significant chance of succeeding on the basis of widely held moral assumptions are the food-and-clothing objection to counting expenditures for later basic health care and the income differences objection to including future earnings.

On the moral questions especially, this is a complex outcome. Yet some crude generalizations are perhaps still possible. When external costs are the focus of a policy discussion, the final balance favors counting all three items. For total costs to everyone, later health-care expenses and future earnings should probably be included, but pension payouts count only in a per capita orientation.

Suppose that these are our working rules of thumb in policy decision making. Then future earnings may often cancel out the effect of later medical expenditures. Suppose that antismoking measures, however, gain less from including future earnings than they suffer from counting later health-care expenses, since smokers tend to die fairly late in their earning years if they die from smoking at all. Such measures almost certainly lose when pension payouts are added, which they clearly should be for policymaking contexts that emphasize external costs. Antismoking measures will then have to rely on sufficient human value in the added years of life to outweigh their added health-care expenses and pension payouts.

Many antismoking measures will be able to defend themselves very well in such an honestly acknowledged framework. Higher tobacco taxes, however, will not be defensible unless they can still substantiate their dubious assumption that smokers impose net costs on others. Without that assumption both the fair share and the efficiency arguments for excise taxes dissolve. Any remaining justification will have to appeal directly to ideals about a healthier and longer-living population, but such appeals are paternalistic, restricting people's liberty to take informed risks for their own perceived good. If such paternalism cannot withstand scrutiny, so much for excise taxes as a method of reducing the consumption of tobacco.[41]

To be sure, the tremendous economic and political power of tobacco companies and other "illness industries" is maddeningly frustrating. As they are driven to accept reductions in smoking among adult males in Western nations, tobacco companies are working hard to make compensating "advances" among adolescents and women and in the Third World. Some greater restrictions are undoubtedly called for—banning all vending machines accessible to children and adolescents may be a first justified step. Then, too, it may be entirely good that surgeons general, doctors, and millions of individuals raise their health evangelism to fever pitch, as long as people are finally left to choose for themselves. But despite all that, the protectors of health in society should still have the strength to acknowledge that sometimes poorer health and shorter life can win critical arguments of fact, concept, and moral principle against indiscriminately health-promoting societies.

Flu Vaccine in Nursing Homes

Where does any of this lead us in assessing influenza immunization of the U.S. Medicare population? Suppose the question is whether or not to vaccinate nonskilled nursing-home residents. The direct expense of vaccination is no greater than the medical cost of caring for the complications of influenza that it prevents—that is, it seems to have zero net cost. But there are no future earnings for vaccination to save, and later unrelated medical expenditures in resultant longer lives, say, are $1,000 per year of life that the immunization saves.[42] If social security payments are also $7,000 per year, and annual long-term care expenses are $22,000, we might say that a policy of vaccinating incurs $30,000 of added expense for every year of life it saves. That puts us into the ballpark of admittedly cost-controversial care such as kidney dialysis and heart and liver transplants.

But what costs should we admit into a relevant economic assessment? Can the essential conclusions we derived for use in calculating antismoking programs help us here?

First of all, there is nothing about the reasoning for public support of medical care for nursing-home populations that requires us to focus on external costs. In smoking policy the primary reason for focusing on costs to others is that some human behavior leads to the health problem at issue; that behavior, moreover, is seen as ultimately voluntary or at least malleable. In addition, the argument for excise taxation in particular requires a claim about net external costs. In none of these respects is influenza among nursing-home populations the same as an antismoking program. No behavior of residents sets the stage for the discussion, so the matter of voluntariness or malleability never even comes up. And we are not in the pay-your-share context of tax policy.

For flu vaccine decisions, then, we are examining overall costs in society, never just external costs. Future earnings are not at issue either, so we quickly narrow the discussion down to later health-care expenses and pension pay-outs in a cost-to-everyone perspective.

Later health-care expenditures are real overall costs. But morally, insofar as the care that they pay for has the same order of necessity and rights as basic food and clothing, they should not be counted. Many medical bills would have that order of necessity, but by no means all—let's say 70 percent. We should count only the remainder in our cost assessment: here, $300 of the $1,000 per year that people who live longer are likely to incur.

Nursing-home expenses are a middle case in this respect, but again we see the bulk of them as essential. For one thing, unlike more advanced or high-tech care in hospitals, they reflect a kind of basic living expense. Let's then count only $5,000 of their $22,000 in our assessment.

The $7,000 of additional social security pension benefits are not real costs in an aggregate social cost context, but they are from a per capita perspective. It is hard to say which is the proper perspective, so let's split that one in half: $3,500. The "I've paid for them" objection does not apply, and the pensions-as-rights argument is problematic.

We thus end up with an assessment of an $8,800 additional cost per year of life for this hypothetical case. Most people are probably relieved by this figure—relieved to hear that most of the prospective $30,000-per-year-of-life costs for flu vaccine for the elderly has been excluded. The $8,800 per year of life saved looks like a reasonably good buy.

Disturbingly, though, the above considerations are not really the end of the matter. Many people may still look at their long-run options for later years of life in such a way that even if little of that $30,000 potential cost gets counted in cost assessment as we have thought it out so far, much of the excluded remainder comes back into decision making anyhow. For one thing, people who think through the whole combination of medical care, long-term care, and pension costs for their own older years will probably take more of a per capita perspective on the matter, so that all of the $7,000 pension costs will get counted. They also know that eventually all of the $23,000 for medical care and long-term nursing-home care attributable to lifesaving flu vaccine comes out of scarce funds that could be devoted to other things in their individual and collective lives. They might very well decide that something like flu vaccine for the stage of life in which they are in a nursing home, though a perfectly good and laudable use of resources in itself, is not of high enough priority compared to competing needs in their overall life. It is not at all clear that they will do this, but they might.

If people really did express such priorities, and did so knowledgeably, would we finally want to fasten onto the apparent bargain figure of $8,800 and insist that they have to fund immunization for nursing home flu? I doubt that there is that much controlling power in even the most sophisticated economic assessments.

NOTES

1. Woody Allen, *Love and Death* (film).
2. This is the focus of the well-known "discounted future earnings" or "human capital" method for assessing the monetary value of life. To be sure, this is no longer regarded by many economists as an adequate method for assessing the value of life, but I suspect it has fallen from grace much more for what it does not include than for what it does. See Chapter 3, note 4.
3. Ravenholt (1985).
4. Leu and Schaub (1983), p. 1910, using calculations without discounting. I have lumped into the figure for typical smokers a separate category they use: "nonsmoking smoker-types." Thompson and Forbes (1985) reject the populationwide cost framework they say Leu and Schaub used in that study and recommend an annual per capita method. Leu and Schaub (1985) reply that they primarily used a lifetime per capita model and add new data for their contention that nonsmokers create higher health-care costs for smokers than smokers do for nonsmokers, despite smokers' lower lifetime tax and premium contributions. Thompson and Forbes (1986) respond that an annual per capita method is preferable but give no reason, citing only the fact that then the data will be different. Rice et al. (1986) regard later health-care expenses incurred by nonsmokers as a relevant item in net cost but then exclude it from their own calculation of a $53.7 billion economic cost of smoking because of specific flaws they find in Leu and Schaub's estimate.
5. Leu and Schaub (1985). Warner (1987), probably the most comprehensive assessment of the costs of smoking made so far, labels the final net effect on health-care costs as "unclear" (pp. 2084–85).
6. The most striking data to this effect are relatively old: Atkinson and Townsend (1977), p. 494; and Department of Health and Social Security (1972). The latter is the British government report cited by Leichter (1981), p. 36, who surmises that in 1971 these estimates of long-term medical and pension expenses persuaded the British government not to adopt the antismoking campaign the Department of Health and Social Security was pushing. A more recent source, Shoven, Sundberg, and Bunker (1987), p. 18, concludes that the average median-wage male smoker currently saves the social security system roughly $20,000 in forgone benefits (1985 dollars). Thompson and Forbes (1982) account for pension payouts but still conclude that smoking creates final costs for the Canadian economy; however, they do not consider the later health-care expenditures of nonsmokers living longer. Woodfield (1984) provides a necessary corrective to Thompson and Forbes (1982), but on other counts.

Very few cost-of-illness estimates even bring up the question of whether to include pension payouts from people living longer. For example, Hodgson's otherwise admirable review (1983) considers later health-care expenditures (p. 134) but entirely omits explicit mention of the pension issue. Rice et al. (1986), pp. 493, 499, dismiss pensions as a costless transfer affecting only who pays the bill. Warner (1987) and Schelling (1986) do consider this factor sympathetically.

7. See Warner (1987) and Schelling (1986). Stoddart et al. (1986) end up with a moderate reverse figure for Canada, but they fail to include either later health-care expenditures or pension payouts saved by smoking.

8. The bottom economic line of alcohol use, for example, is probably quite different. It has proportionately higher costs in lost work time, motor accidents, crime, and expensive social-governmental responses. See Luce and Schweitzer (1978), especially p. 570; and generally Berry and Boland (1977).

9. Mandelblatt and Fahs (1988), p. 2411. The $8,000 figure is their high estimate; their moderate-case estimate per life saved when later health-care expenses are included is $2,874 (1985 U.S. dollars).

10. Riddiough, Sisk, and Bell (1983). A year of "healthy life" refers to a "quality-adjusted life year," or "QALY"; see Chapter 5.

11. I am ignoring for the moment a claim such as that made by Callahan (1987) that we should not spend anything to preserve life after people pass a certain adequate old age.

12. I will not examine two other questions: whether any real loss in earnings occurs when a worker dies in a high-unemployment economy, and whether to subtract the expenses of raising a replacement *normal* child in calculating the net costs of preventing the birth of a defective infant. The first is mentioned by Godfrey and Powell (1986b), p. 9. On the second, see Culyer (1985), pp. 8–12; and Hagard, Carter, and Milne (1976).

13. Yet a third question concerns personal costs to smokers themselves. It is for this question that later health-care expenses and pension benefits probably most clearly do not need to be counted, so I will ignore this question entirely. At first one might wonder why a major 1984 American study of the lifetime costs of smoking—Oster, Colditz, and Kelly (1984)—so completely ignored some of these long-term costs of quitting. Only thus could it end up with its sobering conclusion: heavy smoking creates a $56,000 average lifetime cost of illness for a forty- to forty-five-year-old man, and the lifetime savings of his decision to quit are $34,000 (pp. 121–22). The clue to their omission is their explicit hope for the study: that smokers who realize their large personal lifetime illness costs from smoking will quit.

14. These figures are my own extrapolation from the literature. To my knowledge the major studies do not arrive at a cost figure per year of life saved. Studies of the long-term net costs of smoking such as Atkinson and Townsend (1977) or Leu and Schaub (1983) do not relate those costs directly to life-year benefits, and studies that estimate the number of lives or life years saved by a program do not bring in costs.

15. Many people have made this point, among them Leu and Schaub (1983), pp. 1912–13; Tullock (1985); and Warner (1987).

16. Economists are more likely to say *income* here, not *resource,* confining the latter to more basic ingredients such as land, labor, capital, and entrepreneurial ability. I will often use *resource* in the current, more colloquial sense.

17. *Seattle Times,* June 7, 1984, p. A25. Koop's goal of a smokeless society by the year 2000 is hardly a lone crusade. The American Medical Association House of Delegates is on record as seeking the same; *Seattle Times,* June 19, 1986, p. A8. For the AMA's position against cigarette advertising, see American Medical Association Board of Trustees (1986).

18. Two unusually helpful studies on children's access to cigarettes are DiFranza et al. (1987) and Leventhal, Glynn, and Fleming (1987).

19. On the first count, see Godfrey and Powell (1986a), p. 14. For the other factors, see the work of economist Gary Becker, e.g., Becker and Stigler (1977). To be "rational" an

addict need not approve of the fact that he or she has enhanced pleasures, greater with-drawal costs, and a higher discount rate than others; he or she only needs to claim that given those personality characteristics, the rational thing to do is to continue smoking.

20. Warner (1985), especially pp. 387–88. See also Warner et al. (1986) and Arbogast (1986).

21. The power of taxes to reduce smoking is documented in Warner (1986). But because of concerns about the fair distribution of benefits and burdens, a matter that taxation always raises, one cannot justify excise taxes simply by the relative inelasticity of demand that makes them convenient revenue-raising devices. Other justifications involve paternalism, which I want to avoid.

22. This claim is obviously controversial. I would argue that most people would agree with it if the "ultimately" aspect is taken seriously.

23. We need to be careful about what has been said and not said in the literature about tobacco taxes. Leu and Schaub (1983) p. 1913, disavow drawing any conclusion against special tobacco taxes from the factual claim for which they argue, that smokers have lower lifetime medical care expenditures; smokers, they surmise, might contribute less to health insurance funds in their fewer earning years and create other externalities such as sickness benefits. Atkinson and Townsend (1977) take sickness and widow benefit externalities of smoking into account and still conclude that smokers create no net external cost; they include what Leu and Schaub fail to mention, the higher pension benefits of nonsmokers who live longer. Wright (1986) explicitly takes smokers' and nonsmokers' contributions to Medicare's hospital insurance fund into account and concludes that the present discounted cost just to Medicare of each person who quits smoking is somewhere between $226 and $2,745; there may, of course, be other problems with her analysis.

24. At least anything that would encourage "ghettos for smokers" and not impose dis-tasteful smoke on nonsmokers. I owe the "ghettos" qualification to A. J. Culyer. Albert Weale voiced to me the general problem here.

25. Russell (1986), pp. 35–36. On p. 118, she also warns against double-counting. Later (p. 72) she delineates three factors in her notion of total health effects: "the added years of life expected from treatment . . . plus improvements in health during years that would have been lived anyway . . . minus any deterioration in health because of the side effects of treatment."

26. At least it is in the extensive philosophical literature on the matter, e.g., Bennett (1985). For a defense of the now generally minority view that the distinction is morally relevant, see Nagel (1985). Another less philosophical explanation of Russell's distinction here may be possible. Economists wisely realize that they cannot assess all economic effects of a decision, so they use abstract models of how certain things vary when certain other things change, holding all other things constant. This is not to say that Russell is drawing her line correctly if we really do know how later health-care expenses and pension payouts vary, but it may explain why economists are not averse to excluding certain costs from their calculations.

27. I will loosely use the term *future earnings,* but I will always assume that we discount these back to present value, which is commonplace among economists.

28. Russell (1986), p. 36.

29. That is, QALYs; see Chapter 5.

30. Deriving people's monetary valuation of life from what they are in some sense willing to pay to reduce risk to life; see the beginning of Chapter 3. I do not imply that any of the computations from people's empirically measured willingness to pay that have been pro-duced in the literature so far are correct; see further in Chapter 3 for significant problems of principle in deciding what empirical data to use. I also realize, despite what follows here in the text, that economists have almost always viewed willingness to pay and discounted future earnings as alternative views of how to measure the value of life, not complementary parts of a larger whole. I might agree that the willingness-to-pay model is the essentially

correct method while still tracing parts of a person's discounted future earnings back to an overlap with their willingness to pay.

31. By consumption I mean spending which uses up real resources. Saving might be for consumption later but is not yet, though if we know that it will be and it is hard to track as income later, we might count it already now as a part of income that goes for consumption. See note 34 for clarification of the somewhat different notion of personal consumption for oneself.

32. Culyer (1985), p. 22, notes that consumption is now seldom deducted from discounted future earnings because that is thought to take an "inappropriately *instrumental* view of the individual as a producer" for others, ignoring the benefits of consumption for the individual himself or herself. This is undoubtedly a good reason in the context of a method for valuing lives that is dominated by future earnings already. If, though, future earnings are only one component in a wider framework of valuation in which the personal value of the consumption part of those earnings to the earner has already been counted, we should not count them again. Furthermore, the current discussion involves the externalities of the fair share and tax efficiency arguments, where costs to others are transparently the concern.

33. Perhaps most economists do not share this view because they are already using the value of life as a specific monetary constituent in the economic assessment itself. This is not wrong, just not what is done more loosely in the process of using economic assessment in health policy.

34. The notion of self-consumption and its surplus contrast that I am working with here is not directly the traditional consumption/savings distinction, though it is loosely associated with it. Income saved and not consumed may still ultimately be used for oneself, and a good share of someone's consumption portion of their earnings may go for others' use.

35. By *social resources* I do not, of course, mean only resources available to the government but all resources accessible to anyone, collectively or individually, other than the future earner himself or herself.

36. Assume that the tax-transfer scheme does not create serious disincentives to work and invest.

37. In consumption, when one spends on guns one has less to spend on butter. Suppose that the guns are more or less worthless but that spending the money on butter would not have been. One cannot argue that buying guns makes little difference because much of the money one spends helps others by employing them; that is also true if one had spent the money on butter, *and* one would have gained butter's consumption value as well.

38. This choice seems parallel to the choice between average and overall utilitarianism (should we maximize per-person utility or the total?). The latter runs afoul of pointed objections in the context of population expansion. See Parfit (1984), pp. 351–441.

39. Samuelson (1958). I am indebted to Norris Peterson for calling my attention to this model.

40. Of course, the whole program may have been deliberately set up as universal regardless of income, but despite the justifiability of doing that, its universality still becomes its Achilles heel in the current context. Not that the program ought to be selective rather than universal, attending only to needs; only that if it is universal, the argument for ignoring higher pension costs in economic assessments of lifesaving programs is weakened.

41. Except for the currently crazy circumstance in the United States, where a tobacco excise tax may be justified simply to make up for tobacco growers' special subsidies. Note also that taxes on alcohol are probably much easier to defend, for the cost curve for drinking is quite different from that for smoking. On alcohol consumption costs, see Luce and Schweitzer (1978).

42. Riddiough, Sisk, and Bell (1983) compute a figure of $791. See text accompanying note 11.

5

Measuring Quality of Life

Giving up on any life because of expense is tough, but explicitly selecting some people to live and others not to live is morally even tougher. Yet unless we are going to spend the resources to do everything possible in medicine, selecting some people in and others out is as inevitable as life and death itself.

A controversial view in health economics states that the goal of health services should be to create as many years of healthy life as possible. The basis for this view is simply the attractive, innocent-sounding assumption that for all alike a year of healthy life is equally valuable.[1]

It is hard to overemphasize how useful a view like this is in health policy decision making. Should we put more money, for instance, into hip replacements and less into kidney dialysis? We will get virtually nowhere with the question unless we have some common unit of value in terms of which to weigh options against each other. Lives saved or deaths averted are often used,[2] but that leaves us empty-handed in comparing quality-enhancing hip replacements with lifesaving procedures, and rather simple-minded in comparing blatantly halfway lifesaving technologies such as hemodialysis with more curative transplants.

We overcome these deficiencies if we look at health care's productivity in terms of years of healthy life, referred to as *quality-adjusted life years (QALYs)*.[3] Then, for one thing, we can even compare quality-of-life improvements with lifesaving. When we combine consideration of the cost of the respective treatments, the length of the lives they extend, and the quality of life they enhance, pointed and often rather striking conclusions result. For example, we should do more hip replacements and use less renal hemodialysis—since the former produce QALYs at roughly one-twentieth the cost of dialysis. Probably there should also be fewer vaccinations of young children against pneumonia, more screening and follow-up treatment for mild hypertension, and more coronary bypass surgery for patients with severe angina and left main vessel disease.[4]

As controversial as QALYs are, using them to prioritize health-care services is actually a modest comedown from the aspiration to delineate a morally defensible method of pricing life and health. Aiming at getting the most QALYs from a health-care system need not involve us in venturing an answer to the question of how much money to spend per QALY.[5] QALYs will be most useful in contexts where the question of how many resources to spend on health care has already been roughly answered, as when there is a health budget to stay within. We might be operating in the British NHS, in an American prepaid plan, or in the rationed Medicare of the twenty-first century.

But while QALYs represent a way of bracketing the question of pricing life, they retain the ideal of empirical and mathematical method to which economic analysis aspires. Counting them may therefore seem quintessentially modern. One commentator ventures that by the next century the use of QALYs in planning and organizing health services will be "just as ... accepted and central ... as controlled clinical trials" are now.[6]

Should we welcome such a development? I will focus first and primarily on the half of QALY reasoning that strikes many as most outrageous: quality adjustment. After that I will very briefly address the other half: counting lifeyears. In the end I will defend counting QALYs, but I also hope to reveal how the moral unease they elicit is prophetic.

QALYs and How They Work

There is a common confusion about QALYs that is so basic that we need to dismiss it right at the start: it is thought that they disadvantage people with low quality of life. In one respect they clearly do, but on balance overall they may not at all.

To be sure, incorporating quality adjustment weakens the competitive position of a patient with renal failure, for example, in trying to get health-care dollars devoted to dialysis. If the patient's self-stated quality of life is 0.6, he or she would only gain 6.0 QALYs for 10 years on $30,000-per-year lifesaving dialysis; the resulting $50,000-per-QALY cost would undoubtedly give this patient low priority in most health-care efficiency judgments.[7] The patient will more likely lose out to hip replacements than if we measured the benefit in unadjusted life years and counted the patient for 10.

But in another respect the patient would gain by this quality adjustment.

If a kidney transplant would raise the quality of life from 0.6 to 0.80 for 10 years, it would produce 2.0 additional QALYs above and beyond the benefit from dialysis; at a lower long-run cost, say, of $20,000 for the transplant and $50,000 for follow-up cyclosporin ($5000 per year for 10 years), that puts the patient's claim for a transplant in much better stead against other services than if we ignored the jump in quality of life. Hip replacements, of course, also gain because of quality adjustment. Though no lifesaving may be involved at all, 15 years at 0.99 instead of 0.9 constitutes a roughly 1.5 QALY gain from just an $8,000 operation, a bargain these days.[8] Thus, quality adjustment cuts both ways for patients with low enough quality of life to affect allocations: it benefits them in competing for quality-enhancing services, though it disadvantages them in competing for treatments that only save their existing lives.

How does one get any of these quality-adjustment ratings to begin with? The whole business will be morally dubious if some select quality assessors go around pinning 0.6 quality-adjustment rankings on hemodialysis patients. The most ardent defenders of QALYs abhor that sort of prospect as much as anyone. The proposal to count QALYs originates in a healthy disrespect for judgments about comparative need by specialists of any sort. Patients' and citizens' own judgments about relative health needs are the central focus of QALYs. We arrive at quality-adjustment indices by consulting the very people likely to be affected by the resulting policies.

Such consulting can be done in two ways. It can be direct: questioning people with a particular condition to elicit their judgment about the relative quality of their own health status compared to being cured or dying. Or it can be a more complicated, indirect procedure: first eliciting a variety of persons' judgments about the quality of a whole spectrum (map) of health states and from that data extrapolating a numerical quality-adjustment factor (index) for each health status on the map, assuming that normal good health is 1.0 and death is 0.0. Then, as a particular measure comes up for consideration later (e.g., kidney dialysis), we ask a sample of such patients various descriptive questions, using their responses to locate life with their treatment and condition on the previous map. Since a specific index of that location has been established by earlier respondents, we already have the quality-adjustment factor for this particular condition.

Two notable studies concerning kidney patients' qualities of life have used the direct method. Asking CAPD[9] patients, chronic hemodialysis patients, and kidney transplant recipients what percentage shorter life with perfect health they would prefer over the likely longevity in their current condition, one study yielded quality-adjustment scores of 0.57 for hemodialysis, 0.57 for CAPD, and 0.80 for transplantation.[10] Another study also revealed noticeably poor "objective" quality of life for dialysis patients (e.g., work capacity) though it asked different questions. The dialysis patients, however, gave much higher subjective ratings for their quality of life—roughly only 0.06 lower than the average rank of quality of life by the general population.[11]

The indirect method has been used in Kind, Rosser, and Williams's prominent work utilized in some decisions in the British NHS.[12] Rosser and Kind constructed their initial map of health states by combining four degrees of distress (none, mild, moderate, severe) with eight disability states:

1. No disability.
2. Slight disability.
3. Severe social disability or slight impairment at work. Able to do housework except for very heavy tasks.
4. Choice of work severely limited. Unable to do other than light housework but able to go out shopping.
5. Unable to undertake any paid employment. Confined to home if elderly. Able to perform a few simple tasks.
6. Confined to chair or wheelchair, or able to move around in the home only with support of an assistant.
7. Confined to bed.
8. Unconscious.

Seventy subjects—general and psychiatric nurses, medical and psychiatric patients, healthy volunteers, and doctors—were asked to rank six particular combinations of disability and distress. They were asked, among other things, "How many times more ill is a person described as being in state x compared with state y?" Several assumptions were carefully explained, including the fact that their responses would carry two very important implications:

1. The ratio you indicate between two states ("how many times more ill") will define the proportion of resources you would consider justifiable to allocate for the relief of someone in the more severe state compared with the less.
2. The ratio will define your point of indifference between curing a number of the more ill people or some greater number of the less ill.[13]

Finally, subjects were asked to rank all twenty-seven other combinations of pain and disability and then to place the state of death somewhere on the scale of health states they had just ranked. The requisite interview of each subject lasted one and a half to four and a half hours.

Rosser and Kind converted their results to a scale on which 1.0 is normal health (no disability, no distress) and 0.0 is death (see Table 1).

Respondents ranked states 6D and 7C (confined to chair and in severe dis-

Table 1. The Rosser and Kind Map of Health States[14]

| | *Distress* | | | |
Disability	*A (none)*	*B (mild)*	*C (moderate)*	*D (severe)*
1	1.000	0.995	0.990	0.967
2	0.990	0.986	0.973	0.932
3	0.980	0.972	0.956	0.912
4	0.964	0.956	0.942	0.870
5	0.946	0.935	0.900	0.700
6	0.875	0.845	0.680	0.000
7	0.677	0.564	0.000	−1.486
8	−1.028	—	—	—

tress, and confined to bed but in moderate distress) as equivalent to death. Of the states better than death, they ranked only three lower than 0.84: 6C at 0.68, 7A at 0.677, and 7B at 0.564. All the others fell in the narrow range from 0.845 to 0.995.[15]

Extrapolating such a map of quality-adjustment indices, however, is only the first stage. To assign an adjustment factor (index) to the particular state of a category of patient whose treatment is being evaluated, a second stage is necessary: eliciting from such patients perceptions of where they fall in the disability/distress spectrum. The goal is accurate categorization of their condition without going through all the complexities and lengthy interviews of the first stage.

Overall the indirect, two-stage method seems preferable. Both the clarification of potentially confusing issues and the cross-checking of individuals' rankings of many different health states are indispensable if we are to reflect people's real quality-of-life estimates for tough trade-off decisions. The mind nearly boggles at the complexity of the questions and possible responses involved; as a practical matter of fact those are probably just too complex to be handled well with each category of patients directly who come up for priority assessment.

Obviously there are objectionable ways in which either method could be executed. Rosser and Kind constructed their original map from laudably detailed interviews that included several crucial clarifications—for example, that subjects' responses would be used to establish resource allocation priorities for what might turn out to be their own treatments. Despite that detail, however, their sample was relatively small (seventy) and contained certain unfortunate imbalances. Only six of the seventy participants were manual workers, forty were professionals, and not even half had had experience with serious pain or illness.[16]

But theoretically, at least, those are relative, reparable details.[17] Our central moral concern about quality adjustment goes deeper. Do the questions we ask permit us to use QALYs to subsequently deny care that sometimes makes all the difference in the world to people? Do the answers people give constitute any semblance of consent to the priorities thus generated?

Comparative Quality and Life Itself

The moral argument for QALYs rests heavily on the claim that it is people themselves who quality rank their own lives. If this is correct, QALYs may rebuff all references to alleged analogies such as Nazi euthanasia programs in which some people judged the very lives of others. The underlying argument for QALYs is that they represent people's own judgment about how to allocate resources.

That would be a strong moral case for QALYs, but have people really ranked their own lives this way? Suppose one has expressed a preference for a shorter, healthier life over a longer, less healthy one. If one has only made that comparison between two versions of life, both for oneself, has one consented to anyone saving the shorter but healthier life of *one* person rather than the longer, lower quality of *another?* Has one said that it is better that a healthier life be preserved than one of admittedly lower quality?

This is not clear. Suppose an accident victim could survive, though with paraplegia, while another can achieve more complete recovery. Each nevertheless "wants to go on living . . . equally fervently," so why choose the one with the "most QALYs on offer"?[18] The first victim's previous, strongly expressed preference for normal health did not by itself suggest that that victim's paraplegic life should someday take second place in a lifesaving line.

It will not benefit the QALY approach to cite the fact that the victim had said that the quality of life with paraplegia was lower than with complete recovery. The victim just never admitted that when life itself is on the line, life with paraplegia is any less valuable to the person whose life it is than life without that disability. Morally this fact is doubly powerful: it not only refutes the claim that the victim has consented to the use of quality adjustment in allocating resources between persons; it even destroys the argument that if we did so we would end up with a world of "better" results. Compared to death, the victim's paraplegic life is as valuable as anyone else's "better" one.

If QALYs are to cut the moral mustard here, people simply must agree to something further when they indicate those initial quality-of-life judgments. We need to examine carefully the various questions that might be put to people in establishing quality-adjustment ratios. The literature on QALYs notes essentially four:

1. Time trade-off. How much shorter a life in good health would you still find preferable to a longer lifetime with the disability or distress you are ranking?[19] (If 10 percent shorter, then the quality of life in that condition is 0.9.)
2. Standard gamble. What risk of death would you accept in return for being assured that if you did survive you would be entirely cured? (If a 10 percent risk, then 0.9 is your quality of life.)
3. Equivalence of numbers. How many more people with a given chronic, nonfatal illness would have to be saved from some other threat of death to make saving them preferable to saving a smaller number of people in normal good health? Or how many people in a better state of illness would have to be cured for you to think the situation better than curing a smaller number of patients in a worse-off condition?[20] (If 10 percent more, then 0.9 is the quality of life in the worse condition.)
4. Direct ratio. How many times more ill is a person described in one specified state compared with another?[21]

Now, suppose that to each of these sorts of questions about paraplegia one gave the same 0.9 answer. For the paraplegic accident victim whose prospective quality of life is 0.9, to which of these questions would such an answer provide a good moral reason for letting the victim die when more QALYs could be preserved by saving someone else?

Ambiguity plagues the direct ratio question. Where is it implied that lives—very lives themselves, when confronted with death—are more or less worth saving? What is meant by "how many times more ill"?

The time trade-off question fares no better. In saying one will accept a 10 percent shorter remaining life if one had to in order to avoid a permanent disability, one gave no indication that one thought quality-adjusted trade-offs between different people's very lives were desirable. People accustomed to operating with the whole conceptual package of QALYs, of course, might perceive that indication in one's response, but that would be their imagination.

Standard gamble suffers technically the same defect. With a certain treatment one has a 90 percent chance of complete cure but also a 10 percent chance of dying, and one is willing to take that trade-off: one is directly commenting only on the risks one is willing to take within one's life. One refers to no one else by one's statement of preference.

There is, however, an important conceptual connection between such willingness to gamble and the long-term use of QALYs. My endorsement of

QALYs as an allocation method would expose me to a greater risk of being allowed to die should I ever be that paraplegic accident victim, but in return I gain a better chance of being saved should I ever be a victim with prospectively normal health.[22] This is the QALY bargain. Are we willing to take it? It is not the same as the standard gamble—the risk of death I would accept to accomplish a cure of my paraplegia. But if, knowing full well what a particular state of illness is like, one takes the standard gamble, say, of a 10 percent risk of dying in order to restore oneself to good health, would one not also take the QALY bargain?

Generally I think one would. It must be remembered, of course, that if one ever did end up in the accident victim's situation and was paraplegic, one would probably want to live just as fervently as one would if one were the victim with prospective full health. But if one nonetheless thinks that should one ever be in that situation one would take the standard gamble, why would one not now be willing to look at one's whole unfolding life as a similar bargain? That is, why shouldn't one take the QALY bargain, the risk of being allowed to die as a later paraplegic in order to have a greater chance of being saved for good health? The answer may not be entirely obvious, but willingness to take a standard gamble sets much more precedent for QALY bargains than responses to either time trade-off or direct ratio questions ever do. Both the QALY bargain and the standard gamble pose explicit risk-of-death choices.

The fact that people have ranked a certain state of illness as quality 0.9 using the standard gamble, however, does not necessarily mean that we may just presume their consent to using QALYs for allocating lifesaving resources. Presumed consent carries moral weight only when there is good reason for not having obtained people's actual consent to the bargain in question.[23] If we are going to all the length of complex questionnaires and four-hour interviews to set up our initial map of quality adjustments, we can certainly put in other questions that explicitly concern their use in lifesaving allocation decisions. Better than standard gamble would be equivalence of numbers, whereby trade-offs between different people's lives are clear. Best of all would be explicit QALY bargain questions.[24]

Without some such explicit link between the questions used to establish quality indices and the allocations generated by QALYs, QALYs will remain persistently suspicious. But if either explicit equivalence or QALY bargain questions are used to supplement the others, the moral case for using quality-of-life adjustments starts to build real momentum.[25] With such elements indicating consent to competitive quality adjustment of one's own life, QALY-counting methods at their very foundations begin to respect people's dignity and autonomy.

Hip Replacements versus Dialysis

So far we have only considered the sort of case in which very lives compete against each other. The essential moral pitfall here is clear: relatively low-quality life can mean as much to a person faced with death as high-quality life. I have argued, however, that with the use of appropriate, explicit questions in establishing adjustments indices, counting QALYs to determine who gets lifesaving care begins to receive moral justification.

Counting QALYs, however, generates more drastic implications than just lifesaving trade-offs. One of the more striking is that hip replacements, for example, which do not save lives at all, should come before lifesaving hemodialysis. It is not just the relatively low expense of hip replacements ($8,000, to last 10 to 15 years) compared to the expense of dialysis ($30,000 per year) that gives them their QALY edge. Absolutely crucial are two other conceptual ingredients: estimating that hip replacements significantly improve quality of life and placing that improvement on the same scale as life itself.

Here we face a problem similar to the one encountered in trading life for life. If one judges that hip replacements would improve life, say, from 0.9 to 0.99, one means to say that they should be done before things that improve life less,[26] but does one say anything at all about the comparison between such an improvement (lasting 20 years, e.g., for roughly 2.0 QALYs) and saving someone's very life of 0.9 quality, say, for 2 years and 1.80 QALYs? Life itself looks so much different for people facing death than quality enhancements usually look to people for whom less than life itself is at stake. But if we just cannot say that some multiple of quality enhancements is preferable to saving one life, then lifesaving procedures such as dialysis will likely get virtually absolute priority over quality-improvement services. John Harris, for example, concludes that "only when all demands on resources for lifesaving have been met should life enhancement be undertaken."[27]

The gap between people's expressed values in quality-index questionnaires and a policy of actually counting QALYs might thus appear even greater than it did in the previous life-for-life discussion. It is not, however. For one thing, some quality improvements gain immense significance in the eyes of people who need them. The claim that to someone facing death life itself always looks more important than quality enhancements look to someone with severe impairment is too glib.

In addition, we can close some of the gap by looking at what people imply they are willing to risk. With a time trade-off response, to be sure, one is only saying that one would trade a longer time with worse health for a shorter time with better—no risk is involved. The standard gamble, however, explicitly speaks to risk. With such a gamble as precedent, can we not guess what risk one would also be willing to take regarding possible quality-enhancement/ lifesaving trade-offs? To buy this part of the QALY bargain, one has to risk turning out to be one of the kidney failure victims not saved with dialysis in return for the greater chance of being someone who gets a hip replaced.[28] If one is willing to take some standard gamble (a 10 percent chance of dying, say, to have one's hip fixed), would one not also be likely to take this QALY bargain?

Still, the standard gamble and QALY bargain are not strictly the same. Just as with saving higher- versus lower-quality lives, here, too, we ought to put a more explicit QALY bargain question to respondents than any standard gamble question by itself. We should ask some explicit quality-enhancement/life-saving trade-off questions in getting our initial map.[29] We come back to the same larger point: QALY-maximizing policies can preserve respect for individual patients through the prior consent of the people those policies affect.

Before we agree to this part of the QALY bargain, though, we should understand the alternatives. Perhaps the simplest would say with Harris that all demands for lifesaving have to be met before any life-improvement therapies are undertaken. That immediately creates a dilemma in defining *lifesaving*. A broad definition will only require that a person's chances of dying be high without the therapy in question—but how high? Furthermore, does a treatment count as lifesaving no matter how little it may reduce those chances of dying? If we keep *lifesaving* broad in both of these respects, we will be giving absolute priority over quality improvement to procedures that only give a certain chance of reducing a less than certain prospect of death. Almost anyone who tries to live with such a policy for any length of time, I submit, will think that it throws too much money after too little gain in longevity. When we really come down to it, we just are willing to take our chances of not having all the stops pulled out whenever circumstances hint that life is at stake. The reaction here is part of a general pattern: we are willing to take some chances with life itself in order to have significantly more resources for other things. Hip replacements may be one of those things.

Suppose, on the other hand, that we interpret *lifesaving* more narrowly, confining it intuitively to cases such as kidney dialysis—virtual certainty of dying much sooner without a treatment than with it. If we have already rejected absolute priority for lifesaving broadly construed, why would we not willingly take some risks ahead of time and reject absolute priority for lifesaving narrowly construed? We would want to know, of course, what principle might take its place. Obviously the principle of maximizing QALYs could be one; it might be particularly enticing in holding out health improvement and additional life years, not just good things in general, as compensating benefits.

Nonetheless, in all of this critics of QALYs retain an important point: we hesitate more to let quality diminish the value of life for situations where we face certain death than we do for other circumstances. We will probably temper the degree of quality adjustment we think appropriate for clearly, immediately life-or-death situations. We are willing to risk life itself, but probably not to the extent of using a mechanical version of QALY calculations in which a certain kind of life is assumed always to have the same relative value regardless of circumstance.

Hip replacements may indeed turn out to take priority over renal dialysis, but the use of QALYs must be subtle and flexible, not mechanical. Only then will they reflect what we would really agree to.[30]

Whom Must We Question?

In assessing quality adjustment I have been pressing a query about consent: to what have people consented when they give answers to questions used to establish quality-adjustment indices? This way of approaching the matter is a bit misleading. In reality we question only a sample of people to establish our basic map of proportional quality ratings, and we question only a relatively small sample of patients to place them on the spectrum of health states. To some this may seem to rob QALYs of the moral force of consent: seldom will the actual individuals who get disadvantaged by quality adjustment have been previously consulted.

To most people, though, the fact of sampling itself is probably not very bothersome. In establishing the initial quality indices it would be impossible to approach everyone who might be affected, certainly not in the detail that can give confidence in the results. With a good enough initial sample, therefore, it is acceptable to presume people's consent to the trade-offs others choose.

More important doubts focus on whether we have used the right sample. We might just make it representative of the general population, but then we face a serious complaint: people who are not patients may be more prepared than others to discount the value of lower-quality health states since they do not know clearly how important life can be even to someone with impairment. Those who establish the basic rankings should generally reflect the affected population, but ideally they should also have firsthand experience with serious impairments and threats of death. It is dangerous to let one group judge for another when radically different sorts of experience are involved, and normal health compared to living with serious impairment and chronic distress might be that different.

Is this consistent with what was argued previously about the moral foundation of rationing in prior consent? In the larger health-care cost-containment context, health plan subscribers and voters ought to be able to bind their later possible lives as patients with hard-headed spending restrictions. But while it is acceptable that actual patients thus get momentarily disenfranchised, it is extremely important for subscribers beforehand to imagine and understand as vividly and as accurately as possible the later states of illness in which they might end up shortchanged as a result of their current selection. In that context there is a natural psychological check on subscriber/voter abuses: people have to live with their own decisions. That kind of check seems weaker in setting quality-adjustment ratios for long-term illnesses and disabilities. It is also undoubtedly just more difficult for healthy people to imagine accurately what they will think if they get a serious long-term impairment than it is for them to imagine what it will be like to face something we all commonly anticipate such as death. Thus, there is a stronger argument in setting up quality-adjustment indices for asking predominantly those who have had direct experience with illness than there is in most health-care rationing policy. This may not dictate using such participants exclusively, but it undoubtedly means that they should be a major part of any sample.

There is another, more subtle reason for doing this. Though complicated, it starts with a simple objection. We suspect there will be differences in the ratings extrapolated from the responses of healthy subjects as compared to those of afflicted patients. The only significant variation in the original ratings produced by Rosser and Kind, in fact, was with respondents' experience of illness. But surprisingly medical patients and nurses put less emphasis on severe states of illness than others did.[31]

Literally this just indicates a narrower range for medical patients' and nurses' quality-of-life indices than for those of other respondents. Within the QALY framework, that says two things, which pull in opposite directions: don't discount saving life so much just because it is impaired, but also don't give as much weight to improvements in impairment. (That is, while quality-adjustment disadvantages impaired patients in competing for lifesaving measures, it benefits them in competition for quality enhancements.)

Doing both of those things leads to a real puzzle. We complain that subjects without firsthand experience of lower-quality life are biased, but in which direction are we claiming that their rankings would shift if they were not? Within the QALY conceptual framework we literally cannot say. If they would quality-adjust things less were they more knowledgeable, people with impairments would get a smaller advantage than they otherwise would in competing for quality-improving care. On the other hand, if subjects would quality-adjust their rankings more were they less biased, they would put people with impairments in a weaker position to compete for lifesaving measures. The original complaint now looks incoherent.

There is only one way for it to regain conceptual order. In charging that persons without firsthand experience of impairment will be biased in favor of healthy people, we must be claiming that by contrast people with experience of impairment will rank both quality enhancement and saving lower-quality lives more highly than others will. But if people with that experience of impairment will do both of those things, then they are in effect rejecting the QALY framework itself.

Perhaps, of course, many people really want to do that. It is precisely this possibility that those designing the basic questions for constructing the quality index map are most apt to forget. They are in the QALY business already and are probably not inclined to put the whole framework up for grabs to the people they question. But knowledgeable participants just might express what amounts to a rejection of the framework itself if they are asked a sufficient variety of sensitively phrased QALY bargain questions.[32] It is not enough only to consult a high proportion of people with close experience of serious impairment; we also have to ask exactly the right questions.

This is related to another larger danger. Critics have charged generally that the use of QALYs allows economists and health planners to wrest decision-making power away from doctors and the public, insulating decisions from wider challenge under the guise of a technical formula. What are essentially moral and political questions about great tussles between different people's interests and rights, it is said, get handed over to bureaucrats to be resolved with a relatively mechanical calculation tool. We need not just better samples; we should kick the QALY calculators off the job and bring their technical illusions back to political reality.[33]

The critics are right to this extent: technical formulas can easily cause us to lose sight of their underlying—and limiting—moral rationale. And probably some of these trade-off decisions are so significant in the values and apparent rights that they raise that they should be kicked up to the political arena. But should *all* trade-off decisions to which QALY counting can contribute? Are the rights of individuals going to be represented better in the cumbersome political process than they are via the consent foundation of a sensitively elicited quality-adjustment map? In addition, of course, one would have the practical problems of handling all these allocation policy decisions directly through the political process. I suspect that in the end we will want some sizable use of QALY counting in health policy, that if we understand what the business is all about, and if the QALY counters are really sensitive in designing and using the model, we will place many of these allocation decisions one step removed from the political process.

The Importance of Length of Life

Counting life years saved instead of lives is not generally thought to be as controversial or interesting a part of QALYs as quality adjustment. In fact, however, it is the life-years dimension of QALYs, not quality adjustment, that is more significant in actual calculations and resulting allocations. Quality adjustments seldom make more than a 50 percent difference—for example, only a few of the above-zero ratings on Rosser and Kind's scale fell below 0.845. By contrast, the number of life years saved by competing procedures can easily vary by factors of five, ten, or more.[34]

The essential issue in counting life years is easily revealed with examples. Do we save one person for seven years or six people for one year each? If we are trying to maximize QALYs, we will save the one for seven. Do we save one fifteen-year-old for a likely sixty years or two fifty-year-olds for twenty-five years each? To maximize QALYs we would save the fifteen-year-old.[35] But in these two cases, should we really let six and two people die, respectively, to save one person for a longer remaining life? The impulse to save six or two gets its power from the perception that the one wants to live his or her admittedly longer remaining life only roughly as much as the others do their shorter lives. Harris calls this thing that each of us equally wants "the rest of our lives" and claims that "so long as we each fervently wish" to live it out, "however long that turns out to be . . ., we all suffer the same injustice if our wishes are deliberately frustrated."[36]

The psychological claim here is undoubtedly correct: the involved, happy fifty-year-old wants as much to live as the involved, happy fifteen-year-old, and people often fight for one more year of their lives as hard as they do for seven. But the case for QALYs does not need to dispute this psychological claim. What is debatable is the moral claim that all persons therefore suffer the same injustice if they die because equal desires would thereby be frustrated.

Other moral factors than the equal desire to live are operating in these length-of-life trade-offs. One is some version of equality or equal opportunity. Like QALYs—only more radically—equality emphasizes the inadequacy of saving simply the greatest number of lives. Why should the foremost condition of all the other good things in life—time in life—not be the first thing distributed equally among people? Equality presses hard toward some notion such as the "right to a minimal age first."[37] That is no magic age; the point is just that, picking any particular age, people should be helped to live to it before others (even larger numbers of others) are helped to live longer. A right to a minimal age thus tips even more strongly toward saving younger people than does maximizing QALYs.[38] Counting life years can thus be thought of as a rather moderate, crude moral compromise between the roughly equal desires of people to continue to live on the one hand, and the right to a minimal age first on the other.

Harris also considers this tussle between equal opportunity and equally wanting to live "the rest of our lives," but he comes down squarely against focusing on life years: "where two individuals both equally wish to go on living for as long as possible, our duty to respect this wish is paramount."[39] Insofar as the contest is between equality on the one hand and autonomous desire on the other, life years indeed might lose out. If free and equal people decide to set aside some of the demands of equality, why should we not respect their choice?

But life years have a lot more in their favor. Thinking merely in terms of the desire to live "the rest of our lives" is a terribly narrow perspective on the autonomous choice of people wanting to live. At the moment death threatens, it probably is psychologically correct to say that one wants as fervently to live when one has five years left as when one has fifty. But that leaves out the capacity to stand back from one's immediate desires at any particular moment and make other judgments about things of value in one's life. When we do that, don't we see more value in living fifty additional years than merely living five?[40] One thinks of all the things in life that one values—for whatever reason, desires or otherwise—and one has to realize that time in life is a major factor in life's overall value. Most good things take time, after all, so how could time in life not be an important, overarching value?

The critics' point is partially correct. Because of a variety of factors, including admittedly equal desires to live when life is on the line, we do not think that fifty more years of life are ten times more valuable than five. Surely, however, people do not limit the psychological sources of the value they think their lives have to some very small set of desires at single points in time—that would just be immaturity. QALYs have to be partially right in counting time in life, not just lives saved. Only a correction is in order: a life segment's value does not vary arithmetically with its length in years. Here, as in other respects, QALYs must not be used merely mechanically to crank out allocations.

Undoubtedly much current resistance to QALYs simply misunderstands them, and that must be maddening to their defenders. But without a base of more direct, QALY bargain questions to establish initial quality indices, and without complex adjustments of their arithmetical calculations, QALYs will continue to elicit dogged moral resistance. How well they can adjust is questionable. We remain properly wary about their use. Perhaps they will end up as the morally tragic figure on the health policy stage, on the right track but somehow doomed to failure.

NOTES

1. Williams (1984, 1985b, 1986a) has been explicit about this ethical claim underlying the case for QALYs. *QALY* rhymes with "holly" and is the acronym for *quality-adjusted life year.*

2. Hadley's major recent study (1982).

3. They also get referred to as *well years* or *health state utilities.* Kaplan and Bush (1982) prefer *well years* because the term makes clear that that the quality adjustment refers only to health and not to all the other things that can make life better or worse. In his definitive review of this whole area, Torrance (1986) uses *health state utilities* for the same reason; it is more accurate still in conveying that the relative utility of health states, not healthiness per se, is being measured. *QALY* is less accurate on both counts. Nevertheless, it has the virtue of highlighting the quality adjustment and years-of-life features that raise the most important moral controversies about the concept. For an early use of *QALY,* see Zeckhauser and Shepard (1976). There are many later ones, e.g., Williams (1985b).

4. See Kaplan and Bush (1982) and Williams (1985a, 1986a). On hip replacements, see Aaron and Schwartz (1984), p. 92.

5. Williams (1984), pp. 63, 65, views interest in QALYs as beginning with the realization that methods for monetary valuation of life and health are inadequate.

6. G. Smith (1985), p. 23.

7. The 0.6 quality ranking out of a possible 1.0 is close to the 0.57 extrapolated from dialysis patients by Churchill, Morgan, and Torrance (1984), pp. 21–22.

8. Saying that hip replacements improve quality of life from 0.9 to 0.99 is my own hypothesis. I base it on the fact that in Rosser and Kind's disability/distress map, state 5C gets ranked 0.90, and state 1B is ranked 0.995. See Rosser and Kind (1978), p. 349; and Kind, Rosser, and Williams (1982), p. 292. See text below for elaboration of their disability/distress states and resultant rankings.

9. Chronic ambulatory peritoneal dialysis.

10. Churchill, Morgan, and Torrance (1984), pp. 21–22. The value of normal health is 1.0, the value of death 0.0.

11. In fact kidney transplant recipients rated their subjective quality of life *more* highly than the general population did theirs! See Evans, *et al.* (1985), pp. 556–57.

12. Rosser and Kind (1978); Kind, Rosser, and Williams (1982); Williams (1981, 1985a). See also many applications by Gudex (1986).

13. Rosser and Kind (1978), pp. 349–50 (virtually but not precisely their phrasing).

14. Kind, Rosser, and Williams (1982), p. 160. States 8B, 8C, and 8D are considered void since an unconscious person would feel neither slight, moderate, nor severe distress.

15. Mulkay, Pinch, and Ashmore (1986), p. 32, worry that since measuring health-care output in terms of QALYs makes a greater difference the wider the spread of quality adjustment indices, people with a vested interest in the method will unwittingly alter the basic questions so as to widen the range of responses.

16. Rosser and Kind (1978), p. 354.

17. A considerably expanded and more balanced participant sample has been recently pursued at the Centre for Health Economics, University of York (U.K.).

18. Harris (1986), p. 12. I am not sure that the paraplegia example is the best one for discussing the moral defensibility of QALYs. If we think about the matter really seriously, we might not attribute to an otherwise healthy, undistressful life with paraplegia any lower quality index at all than we attribute to normal good health.

19. Used, for instance, by Churchill, Morgan, and Torrance (1984).

20. Used as a follow-up question by Rosser and Kind (1978), p. 350. Equivalence questions are mentioned by Torrance (1986) p. 25; and Culyer (1978), p. 24. For additional general discussion, see Culyer (1985).

21. Used as the main question by Rosser and Kind (1978), p. 350. The term *direct ratio* is mine; *ratio scaling* is used by Torrance (1986), p. 25.

22. I do not expose myself to having no chance of being saved if I should ever turn out to be the victim with the prospect of 0.9 quality of life. The cost per QALY of saving me might still be less than the cost per QALY of saving someone else with higher life-quality prospects. It is therefore impossible to say just how much less is my chance of being saved as a 0.9 patient if QALYs become a primary allocation method. It certainly cannot be said to be simply a 10 percent smaller chance.

23. See the presumed consent section in Chapter 2.

24. For example, as noted above, would one be willing to increase one's chances of being allowed to die if one ever turned out to be the paraplegic accident victim in return for increasing one's chances of being saved as a possible victim with prospectively normal health?

25. Rosser and Kind (1978), p. 350, supplemented their main direct ratio question with both an equivalence question and the clarification that responses "will define the proportion of resources . . . that you would consider it was justifiable to allocate for the relief of a person in the more severe state as compared with the less ill."

26. Less, at least, from the 0.9 benchmark. It is not clear what I am saying about accomplishing the 0.9-0.99 jump compared to raising someone lower down a lesser amount, say from 0.50 to 0.55. I will ignore this comparison in the current discussion. For one analysis of helping the more versus the less ill, see Menzel (1983), pp. 194–203.

27. Harris (1986), p. 32.

28. The bargain involved in QALYs is really more specific than this. Since use of QALYs attempts to maximize the QALYs received for a given amount of resources, one would be taking the risk of being the one person who does not get dialysis (saving $150,000, let us say, over 5 years) in return for having the chance of being one of the nearly nineteen people who would have their hips replaced ($8,000 per operation, for 10 to 15 years each of 0.1 quality-of-life improvement). Or if in fact there just are not nineteen people needing hip replacements to whom the resources saved from the dialysis could be shifted, ten might have their hips replaced and other people also helped with some procedure that was similarly cheaper per QALY then dialysis. In any case, in the QALY bargain one's chances of being helped by something like a hip replacement are much greater than one's chances of being left to die of kidney failure.

29. In this context equivalence-of-numbers questions do not help. They could, but not as usually stated. For example, the clarification in the Rosser and Kind interviews (1978), p. 350, was that the preferences one expresses will define one's "point of indifference between curing one of the iller people or a [smaller] number . . . of the less ill people." To get at the current issue the question would have to trade off one number of quality enhancements with another number of lives.

30. I have not mentioned a very important restriction on the use of QALYs implicit in the consent-type arguments I have used on their behalf. O'Donnell (1986) throws the following rhetorical question at quality adjustment: "What about that Dublin boy confined to a wheelchair since birth?" Should we really discount the value of saving his life because of its relatively low quality? Here O'Donnell is correct. There is no point in time at which such a boy could possibly be conceived to have agreed to any QALY bargains for his life, so the essential argument for QALYs cannot fairly apply to him or other cases of congenital impairments. I will take up the thorny issue of congenital illnesses in Chapter 6. For a persuasive reply to other aspects of O'Donnell's attack on QALYs, see Williams (1986b).

31. Avorn (1984), p. 1299; and Rosser (1984), p. 57.

32. I doubt that they will, but they very well might.

33. For a moderate critic in this vein, See A. Smith (1987), p. 1136. In response, see the cogent reply by Williams (1987).

34. Roy Carr-Hill (University of York) has suggested that the *QALYs* label with its "quality" lead should be changed to *LEADDs*—life expectancy adjusted by distress and disability.

35. Both examples are used by Harris (1985), pp. 95–96; and (1986), p. 6. I have slightly modified the second one to make the aggregate year totals clearer.

36. Harris (1985), p. 89.

37. Menzel (1983), pp. 190–92, refers to this as "the right to a minimal number of years." Harris (1985), pp. 99–101, develops something very much like it in his "fair innings" notion. Brock (1986b), p. 418, makes the same point with "equal opportunity."

38. If the equality factor behaves something like a genuine right to a minimal age first, then saving someone at age twenty for ten more years ought to get first call before saving virtually any number of older people to ages past thirty, even if that latter group represents the much larger number of years of life saved. Individual rights insulate persons precisely from large aggregates of competing value.

39. Harris (1985), p. 101.

40. The same sort of longer-range, prior perspective on one's whole life is used by Daniels (1982) in arguing that health care may justly be rationed by age.

6

The Innocence of Birth

Whether to treat seriously ill newborns aggressively is one of the most excruciating life-or-death decisions in health care.[1] These patients are so utterly, transparently, completely dependent. With no imaginable say of their own, they have been pushed into life with huge burdens already.

Generally we have not complicated these already torturous decisions with explicit consideration of financial cost. In the middle of their otherwise heated conflict in the famous Baby Doe cases of the mid-1980s, for example, right-to-life organizations and pediatricians could publicly announce their agreement on one thing: costs and scarcity of resources "must not determine . . .decisions."[2]

To be sure, costs may affect some parental refusals of consent to aggressive treatment. In American law, however, the issue is then one of parental rights, not costs per se. Particular health-care institutions may also limit the share of their resources that they are willing to devote to an individual infant's treatment. With others waiting by, each of whom would take up fewer resources, providers may decide not to treat aggressively. It would be misleading, however, to say that they are then letting infants die because it costs too much to keep them alive. These are instances of "selecting" life—some to live and others not to live—not "pricing" it: in the immediate, unalterable scarcity of means, not all can be saved.

The real pricing-of-life issue arises when lives are exchanged for money, when health-care providers, subscribers, or citizens decide whether or not to devote these resources to health and lifesaving at all. This may already be occurring with infants, for example, when hospital administrators decide not to establish or expand an intensive care nursery with what would be new dollars for health care. Even in such a genuine pricing-of-life decision as this, however, people hesitate to say that they are really only willing to spend so much to save a baby's life. They try almost any other explanation. They probably turn first to the allegedly insufficient quality of these patients' lives— insufficient quality to the infants themselves. Yet if that is the only life they have, is its quality really insufficient to them? Despite the fact that insufficient quality is thus often a delusion, people still want to resort to something like it because of the moral guard it provides: if only decisions can be made for the sake of the infant . . .[3] Letting newborns die for their own sake may be playing God—scary enough—but it is not remotely as terrifying as playing a selfish and stingy God to save money.

In the current economic and cultural situation, however, even such well-meant moral caution is unlikely to keep the costs of care completely out of our decisions. One reason is simply the actual expense of caring for certain newborns in a hard-pressed health-care economy. For his or her few years of life a Tay-Sachs child[4] needs care costing upwards of $40,000 a year, and $200,000 is not unprecedented for the first year of care in the worst cases of spina bifida with meningomyelocele. Increasing ability to save newborns of lower and lower birth weight comes generally at great expense: the average cost per survivor of intensive care for 500- to 999-gram infants is nearly $200,000—$16,000 per year of life saved. It is considerably less for the 1,000- to 1,499-gram category: $100,000 per survivor, only $5,000 per year of life.[5] Lower estimates can be found, but they are usually per admission, not per survivor.[6]

In any case, cost figures by themselves are only part of the story. On their face they are not that alarming; some may be a bit higher for newborns than is generally paid for lifesaving, but many, because of the long period of life saved, look reasonable compared to the more expensive care for adults.[7] There are other fundamental factors here contributing to doubts about how incumbent it is to save the lives of newborns.

For one thng, some aggressive infant care may improve survival rates without improving quality of life. A probable case in point is early surgery for spina bifida when prognosis is already poor. Without aggressive treatment, the infant will likely die, but if the infant does live, he or she is rarely worse off for the lack of care. Aggressive treatment only prolongs life; it does not improve it.[8]

Even more importantly, an infant who dies seems to suffer little of the despair of an older child or adult, and death is no affront to an infant's nonexistent expectations. If, for a newborn, death and dying are thus just not as bad an eventuality or process as they are for others, then apparently, without any discrimination against newborns whatsoever, we could spend less on them per survivor than we do on others. We would only be impartially considering all the various people we might save. Even if $300,000, say, is not at all too much to spend to rescue older children or adults, maybe it is still too much to pay for rescuing infants. If this is correct, maybe we should ration care more vigorously in neonatal contexts than in others.

Yet what about the original feelings of special reluctance to pass up anything of benefit for an imperiled infant? I will first develop a disturbing and persuasive consent-based argument that these feelings reflect some persuasive moral logic. That will put us in a real box: either we will have to accept this argument's conclusion that there is virtually no defensible limit on what we should spend to treat imperiled newborns, or we will have to deny them the status of moral personhood that the argument assumes.

Unimaginable Bargains

Look at the moral argument for denying lifesaving care in the analogous case of adults. Suppose each person in a community of 1,000 faces a 1-in-1,000 annual risk of dying from some particular fatal disease. The likely one person a year who gets the disease can be cured with million-dollar state-of-the-art care. Since there is no justice in the terrible luck of those whom the disease occasionally strikes compared to the good fortune of everyone else, the latter feel they ought to provide the necessary funds for the cure.

But then people note that they are sometimes willing to risk death from not treating at state-of-the-art levels. They are all willing—barely willing—to pay $500 a year to protect against such risks; they are not willing to pay $1,000. The total annual revenue thus available for the expensive treatment for the one person a year likely to be struck by the disease is $500,000, not $1 million. Why should people spend more than $500,000 to rescue one of their own who gets the million-dollar disease? Saying they should would be saying they shouldn't take a 1-in-1,000 risk of dying in order to avoid spending more than $500 in extra premiums. But why shouldn't they, if they see the scarce resource trade-offs the way they do?

Right here is the rub when we get to infants. If imperiled newborns themselves can in no sense be thought to have chosen savings over safety, no descriptions such as "respect for their own choices" can apply. The problem is not that defective infants have not actually chosen savings over safety. Adults, too, may not actually have chosen that, but if there is good reason both for not having asked them and for thinking that they would have so chosen if they had been asked, providers may presume their consent and proceed.[9] The problem of justifying monetary limits on care in the case of seriously ill infants is much more exasperating: no even hypothetical prior consent of theirs to limitations on care is possible to imagine.

Suppose we see these infants as making some kind of mythical prenatal bargain for treating their future congenital anomalies. As long as the life saved or improvement accomplished is worthwhile to the handicapped child (considering, of course, what the child must go through to get there), at what point in time can we ever say that the child had a significant chance of benefiting from tough cost-containment savings? Never, not even before birth. In the child's straits, what more important uses of the money does he or she have to save for? The savings might even be used later for his or her benefit, but given the huge initial stakes—life or debilitating defect—how many severely ill infants can really be expected to benefit? Any morally conscionable pricing of life is thus cut loose from its anchor in consent.[10]

We could put the same point in terms of removing the absolutely last conceivable taint on the innocence of infants. In contrast to the way we commonly react to bad "brute luck," bad "option luck" is often thought not to be unjust.[11] Suppose everyone appears to have an equal chance of catastrophe—bad brute luck. But suppose everyone also has the opportunity to insure for protection against it. If some choose to insure and others do not, the uninsured who then turn up with the bad luck of the catastrophe have little grounds for complaint. Their brute luck is still bad, of course, but what is causing their financial hardship is bad option luck; they are not totally innocent. Furthermore, if the conditions for legitimately presuming people's consent to risk are present, it may not be unjust to leave the loss lie where it falls even when they have not made an actual choice not to insure. There, too, the victims are not absolutely innocent—they would have consented to risk had they been asked. But note that none of this gets us even one small step closer to limiting the cost of newborns' care. There no actual or presumable choice is present to modify brute luck's injustice. Newborns are thoroughly, absolutely innocent.

Cultural images of infants and young children accentuate this: they are the "helpless little ones." More active images of congenital anomalies have disappeared. Gone is the "changeling" of the Christian-pagan middle ages for example, the deformed child whom supernatural creatures slyly substituted for the normal, healthy infant. In a more sinister variation, defective children were seen as the offspring of the devil, and their mothers as witches.[12]

By the mid-nineteenth century all this had virtually passed. Only so could Dostoyevski, for example, have used the absolute innocence of an infant to anchor his point about justice in one of the great passages of literature. In *The Brothers Karamozov,* Ivan makes his challenge to Alyosha: imagine that to make all men eternally happy "it was essential . . . to torture to death only one tiny creature—a baby beating its breast with its fist— ... and to found that edifice on its unavenged tears. Would you consent to be the architect . . .? Tell me, and tell me the truth." "No, I wouldn't," Alyosha answers softly.[13]

If the eternal happiness of the whole human race cannot justify the suffering of one pathetic baby, how can the modest benefits of containing the cost of neonatal care justify letting innocent infants languish and die?

Handicap Insurance

A way of avoiding this implication has been suggested by Ronald Dworkin.[14] When option luck overlies brute luck, the key conditions accomplishing the accompanying moral shift are that people had an equal chance of affliction and an equal opportunity to protect themselves. Obviously these conditions are not actually met in the case of congenital illness, but let's imagine that they are. Imagine, for example, that we all see ourselves as having an equal chance before birth of being born seriously ill and handicapped. Back then, prenatally, for what level of compensation or treatment for congenital defects would we insure? Let's call this the handicap insurance question.

Unlike our previous attempts to imagine what choice of savings over safety imperiled newborns would make, this query erases any of their knowledge that they will be born unlucky. If prenatal "people" are thus looking ahead only to the possibility of being cursed with birth defects, their choices will probably not be radically different from insurance decisions at later ages when people consider the treatment of conditions that can incapacitate for major portions of life. Undoubtedly they will insure for somewhat more if they honestly and vividly imagine starting off whole lives with tremendous burdens and diminished opportunities, but that will only marginally increase the upper limits on the cost and scope of care. The important point is that if the handicap insurance question is the proper one to ask, people will bind themselves to some limits.

Here the question itself, however, is terribly problematic. Dworkin himself worries about the indeterminacy of choices that hypothetical insurers are called upon to make,[15] but there is a much more fundamental problem. The question totally fails to capture the injustice of handicapped infants' brute bad luck. To be sure, it brings all of us, handicapped and "normal" alike, under equal conditions. But for the child the prenatal context in which Dworkin thus places the decision is not his or her real life of congenital illness, the only real life he or she will ever have. Not even the prenatal context is realistic for the child. In more typical and justifiable cases of presuming people's consent we also refer to hypothetical choices, but they must be the predicted choices of actual persons in perfectly realistic prior situations. Therefore the answers bind them. By contrast any prenatal version of Dworkin's hypothetical insurance question seems not to take real impaired children seriously. "You claim to be letting me choose from a position of equal chance and equal opportunity," the unlucky infant could complain, "but that's a purely mythical me and a totally fanciful choice. Why should I, the real me, be bound by it?"

I think this is the right response to the handicap insurance proposal, but there is some hesitation. We talk, for example, of the lottery of disease, especially in the case of birth defects. We think of congenital impairments as something that we, too, were actually exposed to some chance of having. That chance, of course, was prenatal, and literally we did not then exist.[16] Nevertheless we look at handicapped infants and say things like, "My God, I had just as much a chance of turning out that way as any of them ever did." We apparently put ourselves and defective children back at a common point in time where both we and they had the same chance of turning out for better or for worse. That is exactly the perspective of Dworkin's handicap insurance question on birth defects. But on the other hand, note the different attitude of the closely associated comment, "There but for the grace of God go I." This does not assume any kind of prenatal existence propelling us toward the handicap insurance question.

So how can we rely on the former attitude in an argument? It is reflected by just one of the ways we happen to talk. More importantly, the reality of our relationship to infants afflicted with serious congenital problems is that they, unlike us, have never had a chance to take account of their prospects in making health-care protection decisions. Why, then, must they throw themselves back to a time when they make a common handicap insurance decision along with the rest of us? All of the only real life they have labors under the burden of their illness.

Thus, while at first sight the handicap insurance question promises to be wonderfully helpful, it finally does nothing to assuage basic doubts about applying to newborns the spending limitations we use on ourselves.

The Questionable Relevance of Consent

The more the implications sink in regarding our inability to presume any sort of consent by defective infants to cost limitations, the more frustrated we are likely to get. It seems that we must spend literally whatever is possible in treating newborns who may benefit relatively little. But how can that possibly be correct while other patients are cut off from less expensive care with greater marginal benefits? How, in fact, did we even get started on this line of argument? If infants just are not consenting agents, why should we have to go through all this business of individually prognosticating their best interest and inferring something about their consent—here, its absence?

Perhaps the most familiar version of such skepticism is straightforwardly comparative. If there are greater needs to be met in other patients, let's just cut back on spending for infants.[17] To use that kind of aggregative, balancing reasoning straight out without explaining why we may use it in treating innocent infants in particular, however, is unacceptable. If we reasoned that way for newborns, why should we not use the same reasoning to resolve cost-containment questions for all other patients? Yet to do that would effectively be to reject the claims of consenting/objecting individuals as the proper framework for limiting the cost of care. If I am correct in Chapters 1 and 2, some sort of prior consent framework is peculiarly able to reconcile health-care providers' allegiance to patients as persons with the demands of economic efficiency; that framework protects medical economics and medical ethics from the most objectionable features of aggregative moral reasoning in general.

All this means that newborn options are sharply narrowed. We want to respect each defective infant, but then there are only two alternatives. Either we must work within the rubric of prior consent and accept the disconcerting conclusion that there are virtually no justified limits on the cost of their care, or we will have to see their basic moral status as essentially different from other, not-so-young patients.

The second option is admittedly controversial, but it cleanly gets us out of our bind. We must explore it seriously. If newborns really just do not have the same moral status as persons, we have no obligation to "consult" them for their actual or presumed consent. And there is an obvious reason why in fact they might not be persons whose will we need to consult. With infants we are missing even the rudiments of consent. Admittedly it is seldom in an imperiled newborn's best interest to have agreed to trade health care for other things, but the absence here is deeper. The infant does not have any capacity to give or withhold consent of any kind.

The convention of proxy consent may seem to uphold a requirement to consult the child's will, but if we probe deeper we can see that it does not. Precisely because the child does not have the capacity to give or withhold consent, someone else is required to make decisions on his or her behalf. On what is then probably proxy consent's most favored interpretation, this involves the so-called best interests test. We are entrusted to give or withhold consent for the child on the basis of the child's best interests. This test's most distinctive characteristic is that it gives the interests of a particular newborn the moral power to hold off much larger aggregates of competing welfare; an infant's proxies ought to consent for the infant solely on the basis of the infant's interests, not their own, society's, or anyone else's.

That power of the individual infant is quite remarkable, but it is no more remarkable than the power of any person in a nonaggregating ethic. Yet how can each infant have such incredible moral leverage without the special elements of personhood such as minimal decision-making capacity that drive notions of equal justice and human rights? Why should we not see the best interests standard, then, as parasitic upon background characteristics of personhood? When those characteristics are missing, why should the respect-each-person, best-interests test not fade away?

At this point a common reply is to cite infants' potential for autonomous consent. They may not literally be persons, but most are potential persons.[18] All we need to complete the argument is then some claim about the moral relevance of potential. Either all potential persons have the moral rights of actual persons simply because potential for personhood itself carries that weight, or they now have a claim to those benefits "because they *will* subsequently acquire an *actual* person's rights."[19] The first leads to all the classic arguments against "mere potentiality" as a rights-creating property.[20] The second involves "actual potentiality" for personhood and seems much more persuasive. If one *will* likely become a person, surely one's moral rights are violated if one is now treated in a way that leaves one mutilated when one later does become a person. Regarding potentiality as morally relevant in this way is not at all mystifying.[21]

In fact, actual potential has a lot to do with the requirement of proxy consent. There generally is not a proxy consent requirement with its associated best interests test because the child's best interests are the most accurate indicator of what the child would choose if he or she could. That would return us to the original mire of conceiving of choices by an entity that has never had the capacity to choose. The more commonsensical reason someone needs to be entrusted to decide for the child is simply that the child's interests when he or she later does become a person need to be protected. "Actual potential" for harm or good is the key factor behind proxy consent.

The general argument for referring to actual, not mere, potential gets reinforced by one sort of case in particular.[22] Suppose a community is unwilling to support the high-standard residential care necessary to make a severely handicapped child's life worth living (i.e., worthwhile to the child). Adoption by a private family would also make the child's life worth living, but suppose that not enough families are willing to adopt such children to provide an actual home for this child. Potentially the child can live a worthwhile life, but that is only a mere, not an actual, potential. If in fact the child will languish miserably and his or her life will not be worthwhile to the child, how could the mere potential for worthwhile life require us to keep the child alive? We may have independent reason for thinking it wrong not to provide the child with the standard of residential care necessary for his or her life to be worthwhile, but the example still shows that mere potential by itself does not indicate a right to life.

This, then, is the situation: the actual potential of the vast majority of infants means that they should be treated as if they are persons even though they are not yet persons, but we must not inflate this to do more work than it can in protecting them. Some in need of care will live even if we do not treat them aggressively; if eventually they will be persons, their actual potential already gives them the rights of persons. We cannot say, however, that infants generally have the rights of personhood; if an infant will not live to become a person, we do not now have to treat the infant as if he or she will simply because of the potential. In particular, some infants may not become persons because we choose to let them die. (Perhaps we even do that because it would cost more to keep them alive than the cost/benefit limit that we already use for adults.) If only actual, not mere, potential for personhood can give an infant the rights of a person, we should honestly say that infants themselves are not persons. Thus, we need not check out their hypothetical consent to cost-containment limits.

Most people overlook the fact that this view of the moral relevance of potential is more resourceful and unoffensive to the protection of infants than we might think. It does not put us through the search-for-consent process and leave us without any limits on what to spend on infants' care. But though they are not yet persons, the vast majority of newborns will be, so they must be treated as if they are. Mixed in are those who will not be persons, and as a matter of human reactions it is extremely difficult to keep them separate from the rest of the human community. It would then seem natural to spend on these infants up to the same cost/benefit limits we derive for adults from their consent.[23] Underneath, this is in a sense discriminatory, because infants do not consent to those limits, but it is such equivalent treatment on the surface that the cohesion of adults and infants in a human community is not ruptured.

However, we must still confront an enormous point of alarm about this view. If severely ill newborns are not actual persons, normal infants are not yet persons either. Any normal infant, too, will have rights of personhood if the infant really is going to become a person, but what if he or she is not? And suppose the infant is not precisely because we are in the very process of letting him or her die? Would not the view that infants are not actually persons then allow us to let even perfectly normal, full-term babies die?

The literal nonpersonhood of infants—all infants—entails no such drastic consequence. Actual potential to become a person is not the only vehicle by which nonperson infants can accrue the rights of persons. Another is the spin-off effects on others of denying the right to life to any normal infant—for example, the emotional threat to parent-child bonds in general. Just think of what letting a normal baby die would say about the parent's motivations and how threatening they would be for child welfare in general. People tend to think that any such derived rights of infants—derived from characteristics of the situation not inherent in infants themselves—are flimsy, but that is simply a confusion. Our belief that emotional damage will inevitably result from violating such rights is much more secure than any belief that infants have inherent rights. Furthermore, violating an infant's derived rights is not a wrong just to others who are threatened and not to the infant.[24] Even if the basis of an infant's right to life is the infant's relationship to other people, once such a right exists,[25] anyone assaulting the child is certainly not just wronging others. Once the infant has that right—the infant really does have it, even if it is derived—why say that no wrong is done to the infant?

Thus, the view that infants are not persons does not throw open doors to abuse, neglect, and discrimination. It will, of course, allow us to let imperiled infants die whom we would have to save at virtually any expense were they already persons, but we can still treat them with the same cost-benefit standard we use for older patients whose prior consent generates spending limits.

The Asymmetry of Nonexistence

The view that infants are not persons with a right to life has an unsung but by no means minor advantage in allowing us to explain one of the most puzzling human reactions to birth and death. While we think it is bad that we will die when we do and not later, we do not think it is a shame that we were born only when we were and not earlier. That is, we do not regret the prenatal as much as the postmortem variety of our own nonexistence. Let's give this combination of reactions a label: our attitudes toward our own nonexistence are temporally asymmetric.[26]

But if both death and not being born earlier are no experiences, why is death bad in a way that prenatal nonexistence is not? Someone might suggest the explanation that there is nothing we can do about having been born late but there is something we can do about dying early, but that won't work. Apparently we have the same asymmetric response to purely accidental deaths that we can not do any more about than we can about our not-earlier births. There is a better explanation: death is bad in a way that not-earlier birth is not because of goods that we as persons anticipate.[27]

Now, if that is the persuasive way to defend the extremely widespread difference in attitudes toward not-later death and not-earlier birth, then death itself would vary in its badness by how much its victim looks forward to the life cut short. And then, since an infant clearly does not look forward to the life cut off by early death as older children or adults do, infant deaths just are not as bad as other ones. Maybe in fact the death of an infant who does not yet look forward to life is not any worse to the infant than our not-earlier births are to us—namely not very bad at all. Then it would seem all the more absurd to devote unlimitable expenditures to saving infants while we significantly restrict what we spend to save others. We simply have to confront the larger moral question that this creates. If a belief that infants are persons with rights to life commits us to inquiring about their mythical consent, and if that in turn leads us to unlimited spending on them that for other reasons is absurd, should we not just deny infants' inherent personhood?

Let's itemize our package of beliefs more comprehensively. We would like to do, quite impossibly, all five of the following: (1) take seriously persons' rights to be consulted about life-and-death policies; (2) reconcile hard efficiency with allegiance to the individual patient; (3) avoid utilitarian threats to equality and individual rights; (4) explain why not-later death is generally much worse than not-earlier birth, and take the implications of that explanation for infant death seriously; and (5) believe that infants are morally persons with a right to life.

It is relatively easy to do the first four all at once, but not the fifth as well. Within our larger package of moral beliefs, it raises less havoc to deny that infants inherently have moral personhood than it does to back off from any of the other four claims.

So we get pushed toward a conclusion that is radical but still practically cautious at the same time. Much of our consternation in not finding any spending limits to which imperiled newborns can be thought to consent is misplaced. In establishing cost-benefit limitations for infants' care, we do not always have to ask whether they might have consented. For lifesaving treatment the same rough cost-benefit limits to which adults consent constitute an adequately cautious standard for seriously ill newborns.

Note, however, that if regardless of aggressive treatment or nontreatment the newborns being cared for will live to become persons anyhow, they even now have some of the basic rights of persons.[28] We must then try to prognosticate what their consent to cost-containment limits would be. In these cases a best interests standard will still apply. If treatment would improve their lives in the long run more than would other uses of the financial resources that it consumes, treatment should be provided regardless of other comparisons we might make about cost.[29]

Damages for Wrongful Life

Let me add a more circuitously related comment about wrongful life lawsuits. In the moral economy of medicine, suits for wrongful life are as confounding as infants who leave us dangling without any of their self-interested consent to limit what is spent. In such suits a congenitally ill child sues a defendant whose negligence caused the child to be born.[30] A physician fails to advise prospective parents, for example, of the significant chance that their child will be born with severe genetic defects; if advised, they would have aborted or never conceived in the first place, but they are not advised, and the child is born. These cases require an explicit valuation of a child's life, but here the life is said to have negative value. Limiting what is spent for infant care and awarding legal damages for wrongful life are distinct and seemingly very different matters, but I will try to show that puzzlements about them are related.

Wrongful life cases rightly puzzle us. A child's impairments are alleged to be so extreme that life itself—being born at all—is an "injury." Claiming that the impaired life is not worthwhile is a tall enough order, but setting monetary damages to compensate a severely impaired child for what he or she has lost in being born is the really tough matter. To complicate matters further, if wrongful life suits start to succeed against particularly negligent physicians, we can hardly avoid the fantastic image of children someday successfully suing their equally negligent parents. If how much to spend on an impaired child's life strains the limits of parental gratitude to children, wrongful life suits equally poignantly strain the limits of children's gratitude to parents.

Technically the only circumstance in which a wrongful life suit should ever succeed is when for his or her own sake the child would be better off never having been born. Only then has the defendant made the child worse off. Understandably, courts do not easily acknowledge such a situation. In *Gleitman* the court asked whether little Jeffrey would have chosen that his life be "snuffed out before his full term of gestation could run its course" rather than be born with the defects caused by his mother's rubella. The court quickly answered that he would almost surely choose life with defects.[31]

Undoubtedly the court was correct about Jeffrey and congenital rubella syndrome in particular, but with more severe impairments and complications we can hardly honestly argue that absolutely any life is better than none.[32] In adult cases of the so-called right to die, people commonly say that at a certain point of suffering, death is better than life. Why may not an overall life provoke this same sort of judgment? We reach this point in a successful suit for wrongful life such as that of Shauna Curlender, a Tay-Sachs child.[33] Because of the severity, suffering, and hopelessness of Tay-Sachs disease the court had relatively little trouble concluding that life itself was an injury.

We do not need to ask whether the child would have prenatally chosen to have his or her life snuffed out. The only plausible answer we could broach to that question would require an answer to a more primary question: do the conditions of Jeffrey's or Shauna's actual lives permit us to say that to them, while they are now alive, their lives are not worthwhile? Shauna's terrible Tay-Sachs conditions lead us to say that her life is not, Jeffrey's to say that his is.

We are not then saying that there is anything suicidal about Shauna's current life, either. Take a parallel famous adult case. Dax, a late-twenties victim of severe burns, frequently, clearly, and vigorously objected to continued life-saving treatment during his excruciatingly painful recovery.[34] Now, later, when he clearly wants to live, he might argue that the worthwhile quality of life he currently enjoys has still not been worth the suffering he has had to endure to get it. On balance, overall, he would have been better off had he died. When for a child that kind of judgment occurs much earlier, we have a plausible wrongful life suit—existence itself is an injury.

But if the child should then recover damages, what damages? Here is the real logical problem with wrongful life suits. That the injury of existence is intangible is no particular difficulty; we deal with intangibility all the time in damages for pain and suffering and wrongful death.[35] The problem is worse: we do not even know what hypothetical question to ask to get at the gravity of life's wrongfulness in these cases.

Suppose we asked what money Shauna would take as an equivalent trade for her injuries or what money we would regard as a fair trade were we in her shoes. Both of these questions compare normal with impaired existence and put a monetary value on the difference, but the comparison we need in assessing damages for the injury of existence is between impaired existence and not existing at all.

We might try a totally mythical, prenatal trade-off. If Shauna had held her own abortion/contraception strings and if she had known vividly and in detail what sort of life she would have as a Tay-Sachs child, what would she have had to be paid to be tempted by birth? For comparing nonexistence with impaired existence, this would seem to be on the right track. Now, however, we have an equally exasperating problem: we may be asking the right question, but we have no idea whatsoever how to answer it.[36] Thus, though it looks right, the prenatal question provides us with no rhyme or reason whatsoever for making any particular estimate of the injury of Shauna's existence.

Dworkin's handicap insurance question may fare better. Suppose we and Shauna were in the similar prenatal situation of knowing that we had a chance of being born into an injurious existence. Prenatally, to what contributions would we be willing to commit ourselves as probably normal prospective people in return for being assuredly compensated if we did happen to be born worse off than never having existed? We would certainly agree to compensation for special expenses incurred in caring for our impairments, and we might want to add something for general damage and pain and suffering.

There is even a problem with this, however. As noted in the earlier discussion of Dworkin's handicap insurance question, we are not eliciting the conceivable choice of any actual person. We wonder how any answer derived from this question can silence the complaints of a particular, real victim. Why should we think the answer to a question put to totally hypothetical agents tells us what actual damage a particular child has suffered in being born?

But though no question for estimating damages is therefore really satisfactory,[37] as long as we are confident that an impaired child's existence really is an injury, should we not just plow ahead anyway even if we assess damages arbitrarily? Is that not preferable to letting acknowledged injury from negligence stand totally uncompensated just because we lack a systematic method for calculating damages? We could still be cautious: precisely calculate so-called special damages (anticipated expenses of caring for the impairment) and add relatively little for general damages (general expenses and pain and suffering).[38]

That may be a sensible resolution of our quandaries about the primary sort of wrongful life suit, but for those cases in which the impaired child is still better off for having been born it is not nearly so easy to argue for awarding plaintiffs anything. Some of the actual suits here are laughable, including the 1960s case in which a court originated the term wrongful life and in which a son sued his father for illegitimacy.[39] In recent, more plausible cases a few courts have awarded damages for special expenses even when the child's impairments were not judged remotely severe enough to make existence an injury. Joy Turpin, for example, successfully sued a negligent physician though she was only hereditarily deaf.[40]

The plaintiff's argument in cases such as these is particularly problematic. There is fault aplenty, of course, in the defendant, and negligence is a crucial cause of the birth of the impaired child, so there is some logic in calling the cases wrongful life. Yet no matter how grave or wrong the defendant's negligence is, it only seems wrong to the child's parents. Should not only they be awarded damages for wrongful birth, not the child for wrongful life?

Could we argue that some other type of damage makes the child a victim nonetheless? Do children have an interest, for instance, in the parents being treated as informed decisionmakers about their births? I doubt it. We may tend to think that the child as well as the parents is wronged if a negligent physician fails to inform parents properly,[41] but any impaired child who is still better off alive than never having been born has actually gained by the defendant's violation of the parents' rights.

Another circuitous sort of alleged wrong to the child fares no better. Steinbock argues that

> it is not necessary to maintain that the child would be better off never having been born. . . . Instead we can say that it is a wrong to the child to be born with such serious handicaps that many very basic interests are doomed in advance, preventing the child from having the minimally decent existence to which all citizens are entitled.[42]

But no matter how much a child deserves to come into the world without his or her basic interests doomed beforehand, how can we say that the defendant has wronged the child unless we can say that the child would have been better off never having been born?[43] We have to keep reminding ourselves of what we are emotionally so prone to forget whenever we confront serious impairment face to face: but for the defendant's negligence, this child would simply not exist. It may be terribly wrong for a negligent physician to contribute crucially to the train of events that gives birth to an impaired child, and the reason why that is so wrong could even be that no child ought to have his or her basic interests doomed in advance. Still, unless that child is worse off for having been born, the child is simply not a victim of the defendant's negligence. If damages are awarded at all in cases such as *Turpin,* we must come conceptually clean on what they involve: the unusual legal category of victimless torts.[44]

Thus honestly described, should defendants be held liable? Only one sort of argument will work: construct a parallel to strict liability cases in which someone is held liable without individual fault—a manufacturer, for example, liable for defects in his products even when he cannot be blamed for any negligence. In strict liability cases, rather than leave the loss lie where it falls, we spread it more widely. We hold the individually blameless defendant liable since the cost of liability can be distributed to many others through higher fees or prices. This is also true with a victimless tort. "It might not be fair to make a person pay damages to another whom she has not . . . wronged, but is may be more unfair still to make only the miserable impaired party pay, or do without the aid he needs."[45]

In one sense victimless torts are less controversial than strict liability. At least the individual defendant is at fault. In another respect, though, they are more dubious. If the defendant did not harm the child, why should the defendant rather than the community pay for the child's needs? The final justification for the victimless tort reason for awarding damages for wrongful life is, in fact, just that the community (not the defendant) should pay. Now we can see the real issue in deciding whether to award special damages to plaintiffs in wrongful life suits when impairment is not severe enough to make existence itself an injury. Should the community pay for the care of congenital impairments? If it should, but it does not have a direct explicit arrangement for doing so, the victimless tort route to a wrongful life award is a needed if disconcerting substitute.[46]

The extent of damages that should be paid reflects the extent to which a community is obligated to support and compensate its impaired children. For their pain and suffering? It is unclear. For the general expenses of life that they, like anyone else, incur? Probably. For special expenses, caring for their impairments? Undoubtedly. But special expenses at what level—all possible beneficial care? only care up to a certain cost-benefit standard? We are thrown right back to our previous discussion of justified limits on spending to save and improve a child's life.

NOTES

1. I will most often speak of the seriously or congenitally ill infant or imperiled newborn, focusing on illness known more or less at birth that typically affects a child for his or her entire life. I will also use handicapped newborn, but in a loose sense; my discussion is concerned with handicaps that are also illnesses in the sense that something medical can be done about them. I will not entirely avoid the terms birth defects and defective newborns, though they generally have objectionable connotations; we must not label the child as inferior just because he or she does not fit our expectations, but certainly serious congenital illnesses are defects in an innocent, straightforward sense. I will not use genetic disease since I do not extend the discussion to adults; some of my arguments might apply to genetic illnesses that appear only later in life, but I will not attempt to work out which ones.

2. *Seattle Times,* November 30, 1983, p. A8. For a concise review of the rapid developments of 1982–85, see Weir (1985), pp. 1110–11; Weir (1987), p. 41; and Hastings Center (1987), p. 9. The U. S. Supreme Court overturned the so-called final regulations of the Department of Health and Human Services focusing on discrimination against the handicapped in *Bowen* v. *American Hospital Association,* 54 USLW 4579 (decision of June 9, 1986). The Child Abuse Amendments published by DHHS in January 1985 remain in force.

3. In the highly publicized 1983 *Baby Jane Doe* spina bifida case in New York, the federal district court observed that since the parents' and physicians' choice not to treat aggressively

was based on "genuine concern for the best interests of the child," there was no discrimination against the handicapped. See Rachels (1986), p. 61.

4. Tay-Sachs is an inherited, degenerative disease of the nervous system found primarily among Eastern European Jews and their descendents. Usually fatal in less than four years, its victims are characterized by progressive blindness, mental underdevelopment, muscle softness, inability to feed orally, and convulsions.

5. Figures here are in 1985 U. S. dollars, from Boyle et al. (1983), pp. 1330, 1333. For the 500- to 999-gram category, Boyle's estimated cost per QALY (see Chapter 5) is more than double the estimated cost per year. I have transposed all of Boyle's actual 1978 Canadian dollar figures into U. S. dollars, then doubled them to reflect the roughly 100 percent rise of the U. S. medical care price index from 1978 to 1985. Changes in survival and expenditure rates could put these estimates off base by 1985, but much more recently Fischer and Stevenson (1987) have found a similar cost of $215,000 per survivor of ICU care for newborns weighing less than 800 grams. Generally, also see Strong (1983), p. 16. On the effectiveness of newborn intensive care in general, see Budetti et al. (1980) and Sinclair et al. (1981).

6. Phibbs, Williams, and Phibbs (1981), pp. 313, 318. Note the Lantos et al. study (1988) of infants weighing less than 1,500 grams revived by CPR: only four of forty-nine survived. That kind of survival rate drastically raises cost per survivor.

7. Shannon et al. (1981) pp. 94, 96: For example, $13,000 (1979 dollars) per infant survivor of severe respiratory distress syndrome compared to $21,500 per patient in adult intensive care, when 73 percent of the adults die in one year and 58 percent are seriously incapacitated. Even use of a generous twenty-seven-year additional life expectancy for a fifty-year-old thus saved still yields a cost of $7.72 per day of life for adults compared to only $0.61 for infants.

8. This general claim about intensive care is made by Butterfield (1981), p. 519. The same observation about early surgery for spina bifida is the conclusion of McLaughlin et al. (1985), p. 1591. If they are correct, one of the worst aspects of decisions about aggressive treatment for the poorest-prognosis spina bifida children is tempered: the possibility that without aggressive treatment, the child might not die but will live in a noticeably worse state than he or she would have with surgery. See also Gross et al. (1983) and Freeman (1984).

9. See Chapter 2 on presumed consent.

10. If, of course, the child would be better off without the treatment in question than with it, we certainly should not spend resources to treat. Then cost considerations are superfluous—we should not treat anyhow.

11. The terminology of option and brute luck is from Dworkin (1981), p. 297.

12. The Christianized version persisted well through the Reformation and was held, for example, by Martin Luther. An astonishing remedy for a changeling was to beat or burn the child so that the supernatural parents would come and take him or her back, returning the normal child. See Mosely (1986), p. 354.

13. This passage is quoted also by Usher (1985), pp. 189–90.

14. Dworkin (1981), part 2, pp. 297–99.

15. He worries that it is in principle indeterminate. If we do not know anything about the range of options plausibly open to an individual, we cannot say what insurance decision he or she would make under uncertainty. Dworkin finally endorses the hypothetical insurance question for want of anything better. Dworkin (1981), pp. 298–99.

16. For genetic and chromosomal abnormalities, this claim need not offend those who are convinced that fetuses are persons. For those defects the *we* is not only prenatal but preconceptual.

17. For example, Kuhse and Singer (1985), pp. 191–92. A utilitarian view tries to maximize aggregate net benefits, all persons considered.

18. The easy cases for the nonpersonhood view of infants occur when the child would only "subsist in a permanently unconscious state"—the descriptive language used in Hastings Center (1987), p. 14, for cases in which it is especially clear that aggressive treatment

is not warranted merely on the basis of medical indications. It is not these easy cases on which I want to focus in exploring and defending the nonpersonhood view of infants.

19. The wording of the latter version of the necessary premise is from Weir (1985), p. 1116 (first emphasis added). See also Weir (1984).

20. For example, would kittens have the right of persons just because we have developed a miracle drug that could develop them into persons? See Tooley (1972), pp. 60–61; and Tooley (1983), pp. 191–94. It is often objected that examples such as this are ineffective against the relevance of an infant's potentiality because an infant's potential, unlike a kitten's, is "natural." Even if the difference between natural and human-aided potential is morally relevant, however, it could not make the kitten example misleading when arguing about spending for severely ill newborns. A newborn's potential for worthwhile personhood is no more "natural" than a kitten's; that is precisely why the care of newborns is so expensive.

21. So also the potential of an already existing person can clearly give him or her moral claims on others. Ellin (1988), p. 4, notes that Jascha Heifitz's musical potential gives him a claim to study with an excellent music teacher that his (imaginary) musically untalented brother does not have. None of this constitutes any argument whatsoever for regarding mere potential for personhood itself as sufficient for the distinctive rights that persons have.

22. The case is drawn from Kuhse and Singer (1985), p. 190.

23. Or we might use Dworkin's handicap insurance question, which puts impaired children and ourselves in a common position from which to establish cost-containment standards.

24. Both this and the previous objection are pressed by Murray (1985), p. 1104.

25. I say "exists," not "is extended to the child." If the past, present, or future harmful effects on others of not regarding an infant as having rights are facts about the real world, then it is more correct to say that the infant's right exists than to say that we extend it to the child.

26. Brueckner and Fischer (1986); and Parfit (1984), pp. 149–86.

27. Brueckner and Fischer (1986), pp. 219–20.

28. I hesitate to say *all* the rights of persons, just as children do not have all the rights of persons (free speech, for example). Actual potential gives infants some rights—the right to life and the right against bodily injury, undoubtedly—without giving them others.

29. This would still be subject to independent views of what justice and equality between congenitally handicapped individuals and the rest of us demanded. The point would be that we cannot just regard those demands of equality for congenitally ill newborns as modified by consent from a normal adult perspective; we have to refer to the consent perspective of the congenitally ill person in particular.

30. That is, but for whose negligence the child would not have been born. These suits are currently brought on behalf of children, though were it not for statutes of limitation, those children as later adults could be plaintiffs. They are essentially different from wrongful birth or wrongful conception suits, whereby parents sue for their own losses in a child's existence. For detailed discussion of this entire family of lawsuits, see Werthmann (1984), pp. 109–26; and Holder (1981).

31. *Gleitman* v. *Cosgrove,* 227 A. 2d 689 (N. J., 1967), p. 693.

32. Any number of recent commentators have pointed this out. See Perry (1982), Bell and Loewer (1985), and Steinbock (1986).

33. *Curlender* v. *Bio-Science Laboratories,* 165 Cal. Rptr. 477 (Ct. App. 1980). To my knowledge *Curlender* is the only decision in which a child has been awarded damages for the pain and suffering in nonworthwhile existence, not just the "special expenses" of care for impairments.

34. See the videotape "Dax's Case," Concern for Dying, New York, April 1985. For earlier printed discussion of this case, see White (1975) and Engelhardt (1975).

35. It is not an easy problem, just not insuperable. See Chapter 3 on wrongful death awards.

36. Some may think they can broach an answer to this question, but I am doubtful. What could Shauna do with the money if she is really a Tay-Sachs child, either after birth or before? There are expenses for care, of course, but they count only under the category of "special expenses" noted later, not under "general damages" for the harm of existence itself.

37. I have not mentioned a suggestion that some lawyers might make to fill in the blanks in a strightforward, mathematical way. Juries rather routinely award damages for passing from normal life to nonexistence (wrongful death awards). They also make awards for personal injury—what a victim loses in dropping from normal to impaired existence. Maybe the injury of impaired existence compared to nonexistence is then simply the amount by which awards for personal injury as severe as say, Tay-Sachs disease exceed awards for wrongful death. This would be a completely misleading way of calculating the disvalue of impaired existence, however. Wrongful death awards are only awards for what survivors lose in a person's death.

38. *Curlender* (at 489) awarded both special damages and damages for pain and suffering.

39. *Zepeda* v. Zepeda, 190 N. E. 2d 849 (Ill., 1963). See Capron (1979), p. 81.

40. *Turpin* v. *Sortini,* 643 P. 2d 954 (Cal., 1982). I say "only" not in any underestimation of what is lost in being deaf but to indicate how odd it is to sue for wrongful life simply because one is deaf. Similar successful suits for special expenses despite the presumably worthwhile character of the plaintiff's life have involved fetal hydantoin syndrome and cogenital rubella syndrome. See *Harbeson* v. *Parke-Davis, Inc.,* 656 P. 2d 483 (Wash., 1983); and *Procanik* v. *Cillo,* 478 A. 2d 755 (N. J., 1984).

41. Capron (1979), p. 89.

42. Steinbock (1986), p. 19.

43. Feinberg (1986a), pp. 152–53, has pointed out cases in which one can be held liable even though one has not left the plaintiff worse off than he or she would otherwise have been. Suppose a victim would have been beaten worse by other bullies who happen along the road a few minutes after a first assailant beats the victim. The first assailant is still liable for the injuries inflicted, but only because it was a fluke of chance that the victim would have been worse off had the first assailant not attacked. In the wrongful life context the fact that the defendant's negligence did not leave one worse off is in no sense a fluke.

44. Feinberg (1986a), pp. 173–76.

45. Ibid., p. 174.

46. I am sure that communities have moral obligations to care for such impaired children, but if they do not, it is difficult to see how any victimless tort of wrongful life could be justified. If the community to whom a losing defendant might pass on costs is under no obligation to support the impaired child, why should a defendant who has not harmed a child have to support that child?

7

The Poor and the Puzzle of Equality

Medical Egalitarianism

As we try to distinguish between health care that is and is not worth what it costs, sooner or later we will have to decide whether or not we should see the line falling in different places for people of different economic means. Here we find ourselves baffled and puzzled, in a virtual war of our own beliefs.

On the one hand, does not care that is truly worth what it costs constitute a smaller set of services for the poor than for the rich? If one is poor one will certainly prefer to spend less on preserving health and saving life than if one is well off, even if in either case one is perfectly knowledgeable and rational. People of different means will quite properly choose differently when it comes to making use of statistically very expensive or marginally beneficial procedures.[1] To flatten out these differences through uniform health-care service without changing the basic distribution of income would seem to ride rough-shod over people's preferences for the different respective lives they have to live. Even if the difference in their preferences is largely a function of unjust inequalities in wealth among them, why should the rational choices of poorer persons be overridden? If wider injustice is the problem, why not attack it by redistributing economic resources generally?[2]

But of course there is another side to our reactions. Can we ever rest in good conscience if private hospitals[3] sell dramatic, headline-grabbing tech-nologies to well-off clients while such procedures are excluded from govern-ment programs for the poor?[4] How can we accept expensive private plans' use of diagnostic tests and preventive measures to the hilt, while Medicaid excludes whole categories of even the more productive ones? The matter is one of public support, and the provision we make for poor people's health care says something fundamental about our entire stance toward the less fortunate. Above all, nobody's life is one bit less valuable because he or she is poor.[5]

Thus, when some expensive technology such as transplant surgery comes on the scene, we instinctively ask, "Who will regulate the allocation of . . . organs to insure equal access?"[6] In 1984, Massachusetts's much-heralded Task Force on Organ Transplantation, for example, stood strongly by such egalitarian convictions; it concluded that only if access is independent of ability to pay can heart and liver transplantation be acceptable.[7] We will let transportation, shelter, clothing, food, and maybe even education vary widely with people's means. Health care, though, is different.

The problem is that the combination of these egalitarian ideals about health care with our convictions about freedom to allocate one's own resources is virtually disabling. Lester Thurow describes the three-sided dilemma: "Being egalitarians, we have to give the treatment to everyone or deny it to everyone; being capitalists, we cannot deny it to those who can afford it. But since resources are limited, we cannot afford to give it to everyone either.[8] In the end we rarely prevent those who can afford some treatment from buying it; even Great Britain, with a National Health Service, does not ban the optional care of the private market. But then if we also stick to our egalitarian convictions, we end up in the seemingly insane situation of funding million-dollar-per-life-saved technologies for the poor while we let them live as paupers otherwise. Dare we give up our pretension to egalitarianism in medicine?

In recent years a popular attempted escape from this dilemma has been to modify the egalitarian side of our beliefs and talk only of the "adequate," "minimally decent," or "essential" care that society should guarantee.[9] This hardly solves the puzzle; it only alters its form. What health care is adequate, minimally decent, essential? We still face the question of how unequal we may let health care be.

Poorer people, of course, may already have statistically worse health and consequently greater medical needs,[10] but we can abstract from that difference. Assuming that their medical needs are equal, should the care they get be equal? The view that it should be can be called medical egalitarianism.[11] The pivotal comparision in understanding this view is not between the poor and the rich so much as between the poor and the middle class. Whether someone sells "Cadillac care" to a few of the very affluent is not the heart of the dispute. The more important comparison is between the poor on the one hand and the middle and upper-middle classes on the other—that very large group thought to typify the level of wealth to which the vast majority of people aspire. When they get liver transplants or routine chest X rays upon hospital admission, should the poor get them too?[12]

The current American emphasis on containing costs through provider competition has only accentuated the issue. An inevitable result of increasing competition in order to control costs has been the demise of cost shifting. Providers can no longer easily charge their private patients more to make up the losses they incur in the care of others. As so-called uncompensated or undercompensated charity care thus dries up, Americans will have to face more directly than ever before the issue of providing for the care of their poor.[13]

Already that care has enough problems. U. S. Medicaid eligibility is a maze.[14] As a result, 21 million to 28 million people remain uninsured, most of them poor or low-income, and half of even employed low-income Americans are uninsured or underinsured.[15] A natural consequence in an economically competitive environment is that private hospitals dump uninsured patients or do not admit them to begin with.[16] The real spur to our indignation about this is that all along the government is giving roughly as much support for health care to middle- and upper-income citizens through tax breaks for employer-provided health insurance as it spends on Medicaid for the poor.[17] Note, however, that even if these travesties were remedied, we would still need to wrestle with the fundamental question of how equal the distribution of health care ought to be. It is simply an unavoidable question for any society with disparities of wealth.

Beliefs on this score are not just details; they affect decisions about the most basic structure of health-care delivery. Suppose we are convinced that everyone ought to receive medical services roughly equal in range and quality. We then have in our hands a powerful argument for the unitary rather than pluralistic system of delivery represented by some sort of national health service. At its core the moral case for a national system is driven more forcefully by an egalitarian conviction than by anything else. For something that so directly affects life itself, everyone ought to be in the same boat. Though in Great Britain people can buy out of the National Health Service at their own expense, that is a comparatively small departure from their basic ideal of equality represented by having a National Health Service at all.[18]

Of course, other factors are important in a society's decision whether or not to have a unitary system. There are supply-side considerations: problems of professional organization and monopoly, the kind and balance of care provided, how it is priced (as distinct from problems about how it is financed and distributed). Sometimes supply-side and equality elements get mixed together in criticism of multitiered market systems; for a variety of reasons, for example, better physicians often gravitate toward the upper tiers. Equity concerns may also focus on matters other than rich/poor differences, and a pluralistic market system may have difficulty avoiding discrimination between people with high and low likelihood of illness.[19] On the other hand, a pluralistic system may better implement convictions about people's responsibility for their own health and value judgments. Furthermore, though universal programs such as social security or Medicare may gain much-needed public support because everyone depends on them, they may in the long run lose just as much support when people see the middle class getting public benefits they do not strictly need.[20]

These are all important considerations in the complex decision we have to make about the basic form health-care delivery should take. Still central to any debate in this area, however, is the equality question. Should health care be distributed according to medical need or allowed to float with the preferences that vary with economic means?

Inequalities and the Value of Life

Medical egalitarianism might easily be the controlling view if we had no attraction to freedom of choice. If the shrewd preference of a rational poor person really is for a relatively lean system of health care even after the society has enlarged his or her resources with its support, why not rest content with the inequalities in health care that his or her choices imply?[21]

One problem is our suspicion that accepting these inqualities would imply that the value of a poor person's life was less than the value of a rich person's. Accepting preferences for different levels of health care, though, does nothing of the sort. It only says that prolonging a poor person's life will be worth less to that person in comparison with other things he or she could buy with the money than the same benefit would be worth to a rich person compared to the things that person could buy.[22]

Take the situation where a hospital saves only one of two people with a liver transplant, the relatively rich one who can pay. The hospital does not have to claim that the rich person's life is more valuable when it delivers its one available liver transplant to that patient. It may look as if we cannot escape that odious implication (calling it auctioning off, etc.) but that is because we keep seeing the situation as one in which the hospital is already assumed to have a transplant service that it then lets out for bid. Such a description of the economic process underlying the provision of the transplant here is woefully inaccurate. In this case the transplant is really a service that the hospital creates at the behest of the rich; the hospital is equally respectful of the poor in not creating that service for them.[23] Leaving it up to their choices, the rich person will want heart and liver transplants made available, and the poor person on balance will not. No transplant service would be offered at all were it not for the willingness of wealthier people to pay.

So far this all bolsters the case for allowing certain inequalities in health care, but their defense is not yet successful. Is there not all the difference in the world between a case in which care avoids certain death and one in which it only reduces risk? In risk-reduction situations a better world can result when we develop care for sale to the rich but refuse to fund it for the poor, devoting that money instead to other purposes that the poor rank more highly. But when death is certain unless we pull out all the stops of treatment, don't things change? "Getting the treatment will then become the poor person's highest ranked preference, . . . so there will be no better uses to which he might put the funds used for life-sustaining treatment."[24] If we allow the rich to buy strictly lifesaving liver transplants but do not provide them for poor patients, then we have just acquiesced in a discriminatory pattern that does not gain poor patients anything of greater value.

This criticism employs a one-sided temporal perspective on rescuing people from certain death. In lifesaving cases just as in risk reduction, selling care to the rich without providing it for the poor can be respectful of poor people's earlier choices of leaner health-care packages.[25] It is not that there are thus just two temporal perspectives, both equally relevant, from which to look at avoiding-certain-death situations. If we are tackling difficult resource matters, the earlier of these perspectives is the one rational people will assume. Undoubtedly it is more difficult to stick by earlier restrictions when a later confrontation turns out to be with death; one even knows that ahead of time and takes it into account. But how else is one to see people managing resources for their larger lives? And why should they not be managing them for that, not just for the time they end up confronting disaster? The later "spend anything, life is all I've got" point of view gets diluted by a more temporally comprehensive frugality. This conceptual way of handling heroic lifesaving treatments will not seem nearly as difficult or strange as it probably now does once we get more accustomed to rationing medical resources in general.

Letting major differences in the quality and scope of health care stand simply does not imply any objectionable belief that a rich person's life is more valuable than a poor person's. If we insist on medical egalitarianism and reject letting levels of health care vary in accordance with economically influenced preferences, it will have to be on the basis of some other charge.

Caring

In the larger discussion of distributing health care, another issue comes up. It concerns not the goal of equality but the legitimacy of the necessary means of achieving it—using the government's taxing power to get well-funded programs of care for the poor. Why and when may the community confiscate the justly acquired property of its citizens? Two classic arguments have been suggested to answer this question and reconcile public welfare programs such as Medicaid with consideration of individual taxpayer liberty.

One is the "tax as rent" argument: legitimate taxes are really just rents on natural resources. The formation of property ultimately involves the use of unowned natural resources, not just personally contributed labor. Therefore, if we agree that the poor ought to have certain necessities they cannot get by themselves, there is nothing wrong with providing those necessities by confiscating a portion of other people's property. Paying such taxes would just be rent on the essentially unowned, collective natural resources on which private property has depended all along.[26]

I will call a second and probably more widely appreciated argument the caring argument. It begins by stressing the benefit that everyone gets from guaranteeing health care regardless of ability to pay. The vast majority of people genuinely care that no one in their society should languish on hospital doorsteps for lack of resources. Almost everyone would gladly contribute something to see that this does not happen, but contributing must take the form of taxation to prevent some people from taking a free ride on the public good of guaranteed health care without paying their share. Britain's National Health Service, for example, can then be seen as a national, government-run charity.[27]

These may be persuasive arguments, but neither finally tells anything about how equal health care should be. The tax-as-rent argument obviously does not. We still have to decide what constitutes the necessities society ought to ensure that everyone has. The caring argument, though, may look more promising. While we care about everyone having necessary and basic but almost certainly not equal food, clothing, shelter, and education, we have a much stronger inclination toward equality of health care. Specifically, for instance, though liver transplants may be too expensive a technology to be included in a rational poor person's chosen health-care plan, we care that any such person have the same chance at life itself as everyone else does. An egalitarian distribution of health care "creates social solidarity, a feeling of community, and the nonmonetary attachments that bind a society together. If health care is not part of the social glue that holds us together, what is?"[28] The fact that people care is the social glue that holds us together. Maybe it is even more fundamental than that, the very explanation of why solidarity itself matters.

This argument is entirely correct in concluding that because of the abuses of free riding, taxpayer liberty does not conflict with welfare medicine nearly as much as people often think. But where in any of this is the case for medical egalitarianism? To be sure, caring about any particular person whose liver or heart fails involves wishing that he or she, too, could receive the miracle of a transplant. But so stated, that caring is highly abstracted from the person's total condition, including his or her modest income. In caring about this full, real, low-income person whose liver fails, what should one want? The morally most sensitive caring would seem to involve an imaginative process in which one puts oneself in his or her shoes. But once one takes that crucial step, the case for equality of care is destroyed. If one really were the patient and could control the use of the accessible resources, one certainly would not include liver transplants in one's chosen health plan.[29] So is one uncaring if one concludes that society need not fund this particular expensive technology? Pre-reflectively, yes, this is uncaring, but reflectively it is not.

There is only one way to salvage the caring argument. If it works merely off of what people are in fact concerned about in the fortunes of others, and if in fact people just do care that everyone should have fully equal care for equal needs, then tax-funded as well as voluntary health charities should aim to provide middle-class care for low-income recipients. But if I am correct, that exact caring feeling is reflectively unstable. Benevolence that takes the contributor's initial feelings as completely unquestioned, without any reflective or critical adjustment for the situation of the recipient, is surely morally superficial.

Again we come up empty-handed. The fact of caring and the possibility of free riding justify provision of minimally decent health care by the welfare state, but they do not tell where the obligatory floor of decency falls. They tell nothing about how equal care for the poor should be compared to typical middle-class services.

Equal Opportunity

Where can the case for equal care for equal needs turn next? Other factors may explain why we tend to see health care as special, but they constitute little argument for medical egalitarianism. Let's look briefly at three of them: (1) illness touches on the most universal and mysterious human experiences of birth, death, and the contingency of life; (2) much illness is not predictable, much less within our control; (3) health care is a primary good, something good regardless of what our other values and goals happen to be.[30]

These tell surprisingly little about how equal we should try to make medical care. First, the wrenching as well as enriching experience of the initiation, termination, and fragility of life can be acknowledged as much by people who choose to allocate relatively few of their accessible resources to medicine as by people who choose to allocate many. Second, the financial unpredictability of illness can be removed by insurance. And third, though we speak of health care as generally a primary good, how much and what kind of care people think ought to have priority over other resource uses vary widely with their individual and cultural values.

If there is anything solid behind our attachment to medical egalitarianism, it must be something else. We need to explore carefully one remaining powerful candidate, the fact that health care is necessary for equality of opportunity. In truncated form, the argument is that people ought to have roughly equal opportunities to achieve the more universally desired goods in life; since illness and disability are major, unequal barriers to such opportunity, health care ought to be distributed straightforwardly according to medical need.

A sophisticated version of this approach has been articulated recently by Norman Daniels. He starts with a definition of illness, explains health-care needs, and then uses equality of opportunity to drive home the conclusion for a qualified medical egalitarianism.[31] Illness and disease are deviations from "the natural functional organization of a typical member of a species." A person has a health-care need when care is necessary to achieve or maintain that "species-typical normal functioning." Maintaining it is not important simply because it is necessary for satisfying a person's desires; such a goal would put us back into balancing the reduction of pain and suffering accomplished by health care against the satisfaction of all other desires, and that would trigger the classic argument that poor people could benefit overall from devoting less to health care and more to other things. Health care's special connection is with opportunity: preserving or restoring the "normal opportunity range," the array of life plans that reasonable people in a particular society are likely to construct for themselves.[32]

Of course, the share of the normal opportunity range open to an individual is also determined by his or her talents and skills. Daniels recognizes this. The fair equality of opportunity preserved by health care is only opportunity equal among persons with similar skills and talents. Health care restores that portion of "the normal range of opportunity which the individual's particular skills and talents would ordinarily have made available to him." Opportunity ought to be equal "in the sense that all persons should equally be spared certain kinds of impediments to opportunity"—in this discussion, those caused by disease or disability.[33]

To focus critically on the potential of equal opportunity to support some principle of equal care for equal need, let's grant this account several of its debatable moves. First, there is a fundamental moral difference between disease and disability on the one hand and individual shortages in natural talent on the other. The former ought to be remedied; the latter need not be. Second, the notion of biomedical need requires no potentially controversial normative judgments that already beg the question of what priority to put on health care.[34] Even with these two assumptions, does equal opportunity push us toward equal care for equal medical need and away from respecting the differences in people's choices? I think not.

Talk of opportunity can itself be rather vacuous. More precise uses of that concept involve three sorts of references. We have in mind some goal or set of goals toward which we are striving, a particular obstacle or set of obstacles to that goal from which we are free, and the absence of all insurmountable obstacles to that goal. Equal opportunity in particular then refers to people's mutual freedom from the same set of particular obstacles to the same set of goals.[35] Daniels's explanation of the particular importance of health care includes most of these elements. For example, he says that opportunity is equal not when all differences in people's shares of the normal opportunity range are neutralized but when all are "equally spared certain kinds of impediments to opportunity," namely illness.[36] One item is still missing here, however: any reference to a set of goals to which illnesses are impediments.

Right here the equal opportunity account is caught on the horns of an impossible dilemma. If its point is just that the opportunity to pursue any set of goals is set back by disease and disability, then, though that may in fact be largely true, it would certainly seem appropriate for a rational poor person to adjust his or her level of medical care downward from what the middle class selects in order to balance out his or her health-care needs with other important goals. The set of all goals, after all, is the point of the project. On the other hand, if the implicit goals of the opportunities that health care helps to equalize exclude or downgrade the competing goals that might lead a rational poor person to adjust his or her preferred level of health downward, then we get locked in an argument about why health care's particular ultimate goals are so important. The concept of opportunity performs no magic here at all in establishing a priori priorities before we get to the real lives of preferring individuals.[37]

In response it might be suggested that it is neither any and all goals nor any particular, question-begging, restricted set of goals that are supposed by health care's connection with equal opportunity. Health care instead gets its importance by preserving or restoring opportunity in a very simple, neutral, straightforward sense: a person's entire future potential. Health care is not strictly unique in this respect (witness education and even certain financial investments), but it is certainly different from run-of-the-mill preference. Health care for the poor should be kept equal because it is necessary to preserve this basic, lifelong potential of the individual.

This may work well in classic arguments for paternalism: we keep the child (or the child in us) from mortgaging his or her future. In the context of this discussion, however, the argument achieves little. The alternative to medical egalitarianism features not an irrational child but a rational poor person selecting a leaner package of health care. And major parts of health care do not represent future potential any more than a whole variety of other preferences do. Additional insurance that covers lifesaving transplants at age sixty looks like a potential-preserving use of resources to a fifty- or sixty-year-old (compared, for example, to lengthy vacations in Hawaii), but for a poor person at age forty that item in a lifelong health-care package may not represent potential nearly as much as better housing for his or her family. Again, we have to ask, potential for what, and from what temporal vantage point?[38]

Furthermore, the potential actually preserved by the large category of medical services that merely marginally reduce risk generates little argument for equality of care. I assume that we do not want to become a society that frowns upon, much less prohibits, behavior simply because of its risk to one's potential. Daniels admits that nothing in the fair equality of opportunity account "makes health protection *so* overriding a concern that we may deny individuals the autonomy to take risks that endanger life, liver, and lungs."[39] If we allow that freedom to take risks because we recognize diversity of preferences about the future, then certainly we should respect the liberty of the rational poor person to shave marginal health care more closely than everyone else does.

One further consideration seems sophisticated but is no more persuasive. In discussing whether OSHA—the U. S. federal Occupational Safety and Health Administration—should require higher levels of safety than even those for which workers would collectively bargain, Daniels employs the notion of "quasi-coercion." A quasi-coercive option depends for its attraction on background restrictions of people's alternatives that are unfair or unjust. As in coercion, the restrictions are socially caused, but they are less direct; they seep up around us in the form of unfair social practices and institutions. To hold these unfair aspects of the situation in check, society may restrict some technically free exchanges. Thus we view "the trading of health for too low a price as unfair."[40]

But what is too low a price? For a poor person, would it be anything lower

than what the middle class with their considerably different realities and prospects would choose? We can marshal a whole battery of previously stated
arguments against setting the cutoff line that high. More fundamentally, why
should we be allowed to restrict some technically free choice to preserve the
fairness of other aspects of a situation if we do not thereby actually benefit
the people who are unfairly situated? If people are poor, their reaction to the
proposal to restrict their freedom to avoid protecting the larger unfairness of
their situation should simply be to tell us to put up or shut up. Either we
should benefit them by our restriction (or others with whom they strongly
identify, such as their children), or we should stop saying that we are fighting
unfairness in real lives. Again we get back to a fundamental point against
imposing uniform standards of adequate health care. Why do that when it
does not by and large actually benefit recipients?

In a particular historical circumstance, of course, more and higher standard
health care may be the only politically feasible way of getting additional
resources to the poor. Then in a sense the public may indeed be justified in
giving resources to poor people as medical care when the poor would nonetheless benefit more from getting some margin of those resources in other
forms. But then the public attitudes that restrict the government to that form
of provision are the problem. Those are public attitudes, for which the public
is still on the hook.[41]

Once we realize the wide variations in the opportunities that people desire,
in their priorities among those opportunies, in their desired means of realizing them, and in the risks that they are willing to take in pursuing them, fair
equality of opportunity is of little help in justifying medical egalitarianism as
a fundamental goal of the health-care system. Here again good argument
yields a strong conclusion for publicly supported medicine for the poor but
not any robust principle of equal care for equal needs.

The Rational Poor Person

It is possible that some better argument for a principle of equal care remains
undiscovered. At this point, however, it seems that our attachment to that
belief just can not hold up. In conceptualizing our goals in distributing health
care, why not then simply acknowledge legitimate variations in care with
income? The basic model for a decent minimum would then be what rational
recipients themselves would choose in shaping a system of care for their
larger lives.

Before we go any farther with this suggestion we must address a very nasty
problem right at the heart of its reference to the prior consent of a rational

poor person. Though this problem is unquestionably a difficulty for the model, however, it is not fatal.

The model itself seems to be disturbingly indeterminate. It is not just difficult to apply in practice because we are not sure how rational poor people would actually choose, but it is fundamentally indeterminate even in theory. The model must use some at least rough conception of the fair share of resources with which poor people have to work in making their choices. But what ingredients go into building up our conception of such a share? Instead of letting choices from the situation of a minimum income determine how we conceive of necessary, adequate health care, do we not have to have an independent conception of health-care needs before we know what is a fair minimum share?[42]

This makes the situation appear bleaker than it is. We have some options. We might conceive of a fair share of income without implicitly depending on some prior notion of what an adequate minimum of health-care needs would be. Though I do not work out any such view here, some theories of distributive justice seem to do that. A Rawlsian notion of the largest inequality of wealth and income that still redounds to the advantage of representative poor people generates redistributive shares without any prior conception of particular needs.[43] Redistributing on the basis of whatever share of the wealth and income of better-off citizens would constitute their "rent" on natural resources might also get along without any such conception of needs.[44]

We might also use some independent conception of reasonable health-care needs in building up our conception of what constitutes a fair minimum share of resources but then still refer to the rational poor person's choices with that share to determine an actual floor of care in society. Even if those critical of granting the choices of poor people an important role build up their own notion of a fair share of resources accessible to everyone, the classic arguments for respecting the rational poor person's subsequent freedom of choice still apply.

Suppose we can do neither of the above—neither construct a theory of fair income shares without a reference to health-care needs nor articulate a notion of needs precise enough to shape our conception of a fair minimum share of resources. We will then be at something of a loss, but under those conditions, so will medical egalitarianism.

Furthermore, the rational poor person model will still be helpful as a regulative principle for shaping actual policy. Although it will not give guidance in determining the minimum income share itself, it can still constitute an important allocative check on how much of whatever is provided the poor should finally be in the form of health care. Take any given share of resources made accessible to the poor (their own resources, together with whatever public supplement). If rational poor people would be likely to shift funds from what is provided in medical benefits to something else, then too much is being offered as medical benefits. Thus, even if assistance is provided in kind and not in cash, reference to the choices of rational poor people will be an important conceptual device in retaining a welfare state's respect for recipients' freedom.[45]

Ultimately our attraction to thinking that a decent minimum of health care for the poor is roughly equal to what others obtain may rest on more merely practical considerations than anything mentioned heretofore. Perhaps it is that providers just inevitably fall into the routine of using a uniform conception of good, basic care[46] or that the vast bulk of differences in income between the poor and the middle class seem ultimately so unjust—a "there but for the grace of God go I" kind of understanding takes hold.

Yet here, too, while either of these considerations might explain an attachment to medical egalitarianism, neither provides any real argument for it. The practical point that providers find it too difficult to shift between different conceptions of adequate care does not justify seeing equal care for equal medical needs as ideal, nor does it realistically help when we get to policy decisions about reimbursement for discrete, separable items of care. The sense that larger income and wealth differences are unjust fares no better; that should first stimulate attempts to redistribute generally, not an insistence on uniform levels of health care for all alike.

Many important health-care services should be equally accessible to everyone regardless of ability to pay, but what that circle of basic services should include is informed very little by the high-sounding ideal of equal care for equal medical needs. Attachment to it is a probably more a clumsy expression of shame about society's general distribution of income than a justified principle itself. The consent of rational poor persons is a far more relevant moral guidepost.

NOTES

1. I will focus exclusively on different levels of health care that rational people would choose in various economic circumstances. I hope thereby to be able to ignore much of the argument for paternalistic interference in people's choices. The most persuasive justifications of true paternalism work off the irrationality of the subject.

2. See Menzel (1983), pp. 66–70.

3. I doubt if any private hospitals now in the United States are free of public support, but we can run our essential query on the assumption that they are.

4. For an example of such exclusion, see Spector (1988) and the incident described in this book's preface.

5. Despite all the capitalist ideology in American culture, we should not ignore the compelling biblical reminder of Mark 10, verse 25: "It is easier for a camel to pass through the eye of a needle than for a rich man to enter the kingdom of God."

6. June 1987 advertising brochure for Cowan et al. (1987), a major publication on societal issues surrounding transplantation.

7. Massachusetts Task Force on Organ Transplantation (1984). See also Jonsen (1985), p. 38, where the report is quoted. Jonsen himself, p. 39, says that "we seem obliged to make the life saver available to all."

8. Thurow (1984), p. 1570.

9. The President's Commission (1983) used *adequate*: "Equitable access to health care requires that all citizens be able to secure an adequate level of care without excessive burdens" (p. 4). Buchanan (1984) employs *minimally decent*. *Essential services* and *basic care* are other common phrases; see E. Friedman (1984).

10. Dunham, Morone, and White (1982), p. 490; and Newacheck et al. (1980).

11. I borrow the term from G. Graham (1987), p. 53.

12. On the economically questionable benefits of routine chest X rays at hospital admission, see Hubbell et al. (1985).

13. Nutter (1987) and the first section of Chapter 8 below.

14. Joe, Meltzer, and Yu (1985) and President's Commission (1983), p. 96.

15. The likely number of uninsured at any given point in the year is 21 million; the total of those uninsured sometime in a given calendar year is higher. See Bassoli (1986); Miller and Miller (1986), p. 1384; Blendon et al. (1986), p. 1160; Iglehart (1985), pp. 59–60; and Farley (1985), p. 477. On the employed uninsured in particular, see Monheit et al. (1985), p. 349. *Poor* here means below the government's official poverty line; *low-income* denotes those above that line but still less than twice its level.

16. See Schiff et al. (1986), Wrenn (1985), and Curran (1985).

17. Brandon (1982).

18. Culyer, Maynard, and Williams (1981) provide an excellent outline of the ideological differences between market and socialized health-care systems and highlight the sharp differences in ideals about equality. In his vigorous attack on the NHS for satisfying citizen preferences less well than U. S. health care does, Green (1986) totally ignores this equality core of the moral case for the NHS.

19. See Chapter 8 on cream skimming.

20. Gilbert (1983), p. 86. For related and opposing viewpoints, see Fein (1986), chap. 6; and Sowell (1984).

21. Free choices, I assume. The matter of freedom from coercion, of course, is complicated. See the section on equal opportunity below for discussion of Daniels's notion of quasi-coercion.

22. This is almost word for word the description by Brock (1986b), p. 409, of the position taken by Menzel (1983), chap. 3. Crucially, any monetary figures that the rich and poor may happen to put on the value of their lives cannot be aggregated in any one pot of value since the monetary units represent different things to different people. This simple fact renders one extremely common use of monetary values of life in policymaking utterly misconceived: adding, subtracting, and arithmetically comparing such values from different groups to see which lifesaving project should be pursued. See J. Robinson (1986), p. 152, for one example of this unfortunately typical terrible misunderstanding. Some may cite the potential Pareto improvement standard in defense of such a practice: if a rich person would pay $1,000 for the benefits of a public program costing $900 but worth only $500 to the poor, he or she could compensate a poor person ($501) for the poor person's loss in not getting the program, throw in up to $498 to the government to help defray its expenses, and still

come out $1 better off than if the program's benefits had gone to the poor person instead of to the rich one. But since the rich person actually compensates no one—the potential Pareto improvement standard says only that he or she could—it is impossible to say, impersonally and in the aggregate, that people are any better off at all just because the rich person gained more in dollar value than the poor competitor lost.

23. Reactions in the actual case of transplantation are colored by another factor. There may be only one organ available to transplant regardless of what recipients are willing to pay for the operation. That makes the issue different yet. In my argument here about expensive care, I am assuming that long-range supply is fluid.

24. Brock (1986b), p. 414.

25. Brock (1986b), p. 415, recognizes this, though he does not share the opinion I express in the rest of this paragraph that the earlier temporal perspective on life-or-death rescue is the better one in the resource-use context.

26. Brody (1981) and Brody (1983).

27. Culyer (1976), pp. 89–91. The difference between the "free rider" version of this argument and an "assurance" version that I have not mentioned is clarified by Buchanan (1985). Sugden (1983) criticizes the caring argument on the basis of empirical data about charitable behavior but does not really deal with the argument's driving conviction that regardless of how much one gives or the charity ends up getting, it is simply unfair to allow people a free ride on a public good without contributing anything themselves. On other matters, see the response to Sugden by Culyer and Posnett (1985) and Sugden's rejoinder (1985a).

28. Thurow (1984), p. 1571.

29. Except perhaps in cases of relatively young victims with long years of life at stake.

30. President's Commission (1983), pp. 12, 16–17.

31. Daniels is by no means a strict egalitarian. He argues only that health care should be distributed according to need and in consideration of equality of opportunity, as opposed to desire, choice, or preference.

32. Daniels (1985a), pp. 26–28.

33. Ibid., p. 33; and Daniels (1985b), p. 108.

34. For a critical view of this, see Agich (1985), pp. 3–10.

35. In this analysis of opportunity and equal oppotunity, I am following Westen (1985), pp. 840–41.

36. Danicls (1985a), p. 52.

37. Daniels (1985a), p. 226, recognizes this. In discussing whether the federal government should fund heart transplants, he notes that the acute-care bias any such funding would represent may already fail to protect equal opportunity as well as other uses would. Still, though, he finally gives health care an edge.

38. Equal opportunity does generate a stronger argument for equality of prenatal, maternal, and child care. The unqualified potential of another person is clearly at stake.

39. Daniels (1985a), p. 153. He concludes that fair equality of opportunity does not show health care to be special enough to justify the U. S. federal Occupational Safety and Health Administration's strong technical feasibility criterion (pp. 153–56).

40. Daniels (1985a), pp. 171–76.

41. See Menzel (1983), pp. 92–93.

42. Daniels (1985a), pp. 21–23.

43. For the full theory, see Rawls (1971). In my comment here I am not taking account of the condition of fair equality of opportunity that Rawls places on the inequalities that his principle permits.

44. For the rent theory, see Brody (1983) and the discussion earlier in this chapter.

45. To avoid discussing important paternalistic arguments that one always seems to run up against in arguing for cash aid, I have deliberately not argued here for cash and against providing benefits in kind. See Kelman (1986) and Menzel (1983), pp. 72–103, for lengthy statements of respective positions for and against in-kind aid. Kelman explicitly tries to

avoid paternalistic arguments against cash, but his loose talk of rights to life prevents his view from being of any help in this discussion of a decent minimum for health care. Note that the rational poor person model does not necessarily end up endorsing cash aid in general.

46. This is one of Baily's (1986) major points in arguing for a middle-class standard for the decent minimum.

8

Real Competition

Corporate, for-profit medicine is growing rapidly. Will community hospitals be able to survive? Will financial pressures allow clinics and hospitals to provide care for patients unable to pay? Will physicians and nurses become so business-minded that they lose their ultimate loyalty to patients? I will focus on only one aspect of this nest of problems: not for-profit arrangements pe se but competition. Many people take the two to be the same, for competition and its pressure to keep prices down and services appealing is associated with profit seeking. That the two are different, however, can be understood by noting that nonprofit providers can heatedly compete or that for-profit providers can be insulated from competition by monopoly power. It is probably actually competition that is the primary object of concern in most of the consternation people voice about the increasingly business-dominated climate of American medicine.[1]

In the United States, of course, stimulating competition has become deliberate policy. It has three goals. It allegedly drives out waste—needless care, empty beds, and so on. It also makes us attend to the cost efficiency of health services—whether, though a procedure produces some benefit, some other use of health-care dollars would accomplish more in saving lives and preserving or restoring health or would produce as great a health benefit more cheaply. And finally, it forces us to decide when health care is humanly worth its cost—that is, when we should shift the financial resources to something other than health care entirely.

Competitivists have little trouble explaining that their first two goals will naturally be accomplished if competition is genuine—if the health-care marketplace is truly open to new providers and if consumers or their representatives can see when they are getting more for their money by choosing one plan or provider over another. It is somewhat more difficult to get agreement that something close to genuine competition can actually exist in a real medical economy or that, if it does, it will accomplish the additional goal of restricting us to costworthy care. The typical argument that competition will help to accomplish this third goal involves a claim of moral principle and a claim of historical fact. First, if knowledgeable consumers would actually prefer that money be spent on a certain margin of health care rather than on other things, that is a good reason for devoting those resources to it. And second, in the long run a commercial marketplace for care is more likely to reflect those preferences than either government regulations or relieving providers of competition.

Regardless of whether competition wins that round of the argument, however, the most contentious leg of the debate about competition concerns something else. Most are inclined to agree with competitivists about the important moral role of consumer preferences.[2] Thus, if consumers knowingly consent to leaner packages of care, they are generally indicating something very important about the worth of the items left out. None of this, however, addresses the most deep-seated source of ethical reservations about competition as an organizational strategy for health care: questions of equity.

What Is Really Involved

Though a lot has already become clear since the advent of competition as a major part of U.S. cost-containment strategy, much more will be involved than we have seen yet.

Devices such as DRGs[3] are a mild competitive step for a large government program such as Medicare. Medicare could have both hospitals and physicians directly bid against each other for its business. In similar ways, large coalitions of businesses and insurance companies could amass their market power against providers.[4]

To get genuine competition, the U.S. federal government will have to eliminate or severely modify its massive U.S. tax break of more than 35 percent for the health care of most of the employed population.[5] If competitive pressures currently seem to be getting powerful in the medical economy, just think what they would be if the tax break were ever eliminated. Currently health care purchased via employer-paid premiums gets more than a one-third price advantage in competing with most other uses of consumer dollars.

Competition should reduce not only the price but the volume of particular services. That requires certain incentive structures for providers of which we have currently seen very little. One is capitation prepayment: providers will be paid only so much per patient cared for, so much per client on their rolls, so much per subscriber covered and so on, not an amount proportional to the care they actually provide. DRGs are a truncated, primitive (some would say absurd) version of capitation prepayment; they will be superseded by more comprehensive forms such as entire prepaid plans.

If prepaid plans continue to bear out their currently documented savings but are still resisted by consumers, stronger steps might be taken to encourage people to try them. Lockheed Corporation, for example, is already initially offering only one option to its new employees. Lockheed has its own preferred HMO; only after a year with the company can an employee switch to a fee-for-service plan.[6]

So what has been tried in the United States to date is hardly a fair test of competition as cost containment. Many people have recently gotten the impression that competition has failed to hold down costs; after slower growth from 1982 to 1986, for example, national health expenditures jumped again in 1987 from 10.8 to 11.4 percent of GNP.[7] The four steps listed above, however, show what would be involved in a reasonably complete competitive approach. The full version of competition might have a cost-containing effect barely observed to date.

But in any case, real competition will involve further developments that cause doubt about whether it can be just or equitable. With competition in place for any reasonable length of time, charity care will virtually disappear. Providers will be severely restricted in shifting costs to private paying patients to cover the care of those unable to pay. This is inevitable. They can no longer charge paying patients more than what their care actually costs if they are going to bid successfully against competitors for those patients. This demise of cost shifting was openly predicted by the early proponents of competition. In a highly competitive medical economy the only way to provide for those unable to pay is for the society to fund some arrangement for their care explicitly.

Competition will increase pressures on sicker subscribers toward adverse selection of more comprehensive plans, and insurers will attempt to skim the cream of healthy subscribers into lower-cost coverage. The result is that the likely well and the likely ill will not pay anything close to the same premiums for their packages of care. In particular, patient cost sharing (deductibles and copayments) will become an important part of the total picture. Plans with cost-sharing options will attract a significant number of subscribers—cost sharing cuts down on some of the less necessary uses of care. But such arrangements will also be less attractive to the least healthy people in the population. Plans that resist cost-sharing options run a big risk of attracting a less healthy than average group of subscribers.

If patients are going to receive only care worth its cost, providers will not be prescribing all the care of likely benefit to their individual patients. But then providers will face the terribly difficult problem of whether or not to tell their patients that particular care is being withheld because of cost. It is completely clear where competitive economic interests in this situation will pull: do not tell the patient. But shouldn't providers tell? Wouldn't it be unfair to patients for them not to?

I will take up some of the moral questions raised by these last three aspects of competition: the demise of cost shifting for unreimbursed care, adverse selection and cream skimming, and not informing patients of possibly beneficial care that is withheld. The direction of my argument will be that with the right—in some cases perhaps extraordinary—political and moral will, historically realistic forms of competition can be made morally acceptable.

The Demise of Regressive Benevolence

Medicare's use of DRGs has taken a lot of the heat for strapping hospitals in their ability to care for patients unable to pay. This blame is grossly misplaced. It is cost-containment measures and competition in general that have created the squeeze against shifting the cost of unreimbursed care to private paying patients.[8] DRGs are only a small part of a strategy of competition, a part that would be completely ineffective if the rest of the medical economy was not competitive. Without competition, providers would just recoup their perceived losses from Medicare with higher charges to private patients, and no net health-care dollars would be saved. It is thus hypocritical to laud the cost-containing effects of DRGs while lamenting the related demise of cost shifting. The two go hand in hand.

But isn't this demise of cost shifting the moral Achilles heel of competition? Who can stomach competition if it results in turning away at the hospital door those unable to pay? A powerful case, though, can be made against cost shifting. I shall first note some of its suspicious characteristics, then several things about devising acceptable substitutes.

(1) With cost shifting, unreimbursed charity care is neither unreimbursed nor charitable. Providers get paid for it by the makeup from private paying patients. And the private patients who are really paying for it do not voluntarily give anything. They have no choice in the matter; what they do is hardly charity.

(2) Cost shifting reflects monopolistic power. Cost shifting can never develop in the first place without providers having some sort of monopolistic power. Only because they can create demand for their own services and then effectively name their price can they charge paying patients more than those

who are not able to pay. This has little to do with whether they are the only provider in the community or one among a short supply. All it takes for doctors and hospitals to have effective monopoly power is for insurers and patients to be unable to shop around for competing goods and prices. If they were able to shop around, other providers would quickly attract privately insured patients with lower prices or better services. Charity care may in some sense reflect the noble intentions of health-care providers, but it also reflects their monopolistic power.[9]

Seeing this allows us to recognize how many unnecessary, dangerous, and noncostworthy practices go hand in hand with cost shifting. With its attendant monopolistic power, providers will feather their own nests by giving diminishingly beneficial and increasingly expensive marginal services. That itself is a very heavy mark against cost shifting. What is at issue here is not just a few ill-spent dollars. It is the basic allocation of power over huge amounts of resources.[10]

(3) Cost-shifting threatens the recipient's dignity. Acknowledging the monopolistic power that enables providers to shift costs throws additional light on a long-perceived characteristic of charity care: it is demeaning to recipients. Cost shifting gives recipients the impression that the society is just leaving it up to somebody else to fund their care at this other person's power and discretion. Unless they have reason to be confident that their care will be dependably forthcoming, they will feel vulnerable. But why should they see their care as dependably forthcoming? Experience now with the fragility of charity care once monopoly power is removed accentuates the fact that when providers provide, they usually do it because they have unusual economic power, not because they are charitable.

(4) Cost shifting is an objectionably placed excise tax. The revenue for unreimbursed care comes largely from higher charges to other patients and is thus a kind of excise tax on their care.[11] There is nothing inherently wrong with excise taxes, of course, but this one is suspicious right from the start. Suppose those who cannot pay have a right to basic health care (or at least that society has a collective obligation to provide this care).[12] To implement this, why would one want to tax others who are buying health care instead of using revenue from the general population? Those who buy the most health care are usually those who have the greatest, most unfortunate medical needs. Such an excise tax is also regressive; it hits the highest-income groups the lightest and middle-income ones the heaviest.[13]

Some will say, of course, that it does not matter if cost shifting and charity care are not ideal. What can be put in its place? What likely *will* be put in its place? Competition needs an explicit assumption by society of the obligation to fund care for those unable to pay. In one respect its advocates are correct in absolving themselves of blame: there is nothing the least bit contradictory in advocating competition as a way to contain the cost of care at the same time as one argues that society has an obligation to see to it that everyone has realistic access to a decent minimum. But there is something lame in this defense. To be sure, there is nothing in the competitivist model the least bit incompatible with a societal guarantee of access, but when the push for competition began, what reason was there for its proponents to think that if society adopted this strategy it really would provide such care? Are not competition's advocates accountable for the havoc foreseeably caused by their strategy?

However, this criticism may be presupposing a very incomplete picture of the real options. Let's look at three major ways society could get the revenue with which to fund a more explicit guarantee of basic care and compare them with the cost shifting of the recent past: raising the payroll tax, raising the income tax, or capping or eliminating the taxable income exclusion for employer-paid premiums.

First note that the amount of the existing tax break that accrues to middle- and upper-income citizens has exceeded the total of Medicaid funds for the poor.[14] Medicaid's budget could virtually double if the taxable income exclusion for employer-paid insurance premiums were eliminated.

Second, compare the distributive effects of the various options for financing a guarantee of minimally decent care—cost shifting, an additional payroll tax, an income tax increase, and capping (only capping, not eliminating) the family tax break for employer-paid premiums at $1,500 (see Table 2). The payroll tax is slightly progressive when comparing low- with middle-income groups but regressive when comparing any others. The income tax has the most progressive distributive effects but involves the politically difficult step of positively raising a tax, and neither the payroll nor the income tax option constitutes any new incentive for cost containment. Capping the tax break for employer-paid premiums is almost as progressive a revenue source, and

Table 2. Revenue Contributions by Income Group

Income quintile	% of total income	(a) % of present cost shifting	(b) % of payroll tax	(c) % of income tax	(d) % of $ from cap on tax break	Change in percentage by substituting (d) for (a)
1 (low)	6	6	3	1	3	3% less
2	12	12	9	4	8	4% less
3	17	23	18	11	13	10% less
4	23	26	29	23	25	1% more
5 (high)	42	34	41	61	52	18% more

it also has the considerable cost-containment merit of confronting employees with the true cost of devoting additional dollars to expansive, expensive health-care plans.

It might be argued that cost shifting and the current uncapped taxable income exclusion go hand in hand: the tax break for the privately insured then makes it equitable for society to take that revenue back by the hidden excise tax of cost shifting. That logic, though, is oblivious to the distributive effects just noted: if one regressive policy (tax break) legitimizes another (cost shifting), does this not result in a doubly regressive policy?[16]

Thus, critics of competition simply have to admit that the current economy they are criticizing is only a half-baked loaf of competition, and a crazy one at that. One of the essential components at the very heart of the competitive model—significantly capping or eliminating the taxable income exclusion—has so far not been implemented. Advocates of real competition have all along assumed it to be integral to the entire competitive scheme; if it were implemented, there would be additional revenue for a more adequate guarantee of access. Such a guarantee would be funded more fairly than a weaker guarantee ever is through cost shifting and would constitute a more dignifying structure for delivering care to recipients.

Such a guarantee of access may be politically feasible, even without the revenue-producing step of reducing or eliminating the tax break. Witness the recent state of Massachusetts action expanding access, for example.[17] But if in fact it should eventually prove to be politically impossible to marry an adequate guarantee of access with competition, competitivists will have to consider defending their model only as an ideal, without pressing vigorously for actually using it in the current, historical United States. That would be regrettable, for one reason, because continuing with cost shifting is so objectionable. How can it be right for a society to extract for the poor by hidden and regressive means what it is not willing to provide when all the facts are put out openly on the public table? This creates a very serious dilemma, one in which people opposed to a competitivist stategy do not come out clean, either. If basic care for the poor "can only be enacted by subterfuge and deceit, how can one judge" whether that program is adequate?[18]

Adverse Selection and Cream Skimming

In economic competition, every insurer tries to avoid attracting sicker subscribers than its competitors. The higher premiums required will not be accepted by other, healthier subscribers who can find savings elsewhere. As sicker people are attracted and healthier ones leave for other plans, premiums will rise even more for the remaining membership.

Is it wrong for healthier people to flee groups with more likely ill subscribers? Should they not help pay to support the more likely ill? That is, should they not pay something close to "community"- rather than "experience"-rated premiums? One consideration says that they ought to: for access to health care to be equitable, those who have had the sheer misfortune of more likely needing care should not have to pay a lot more for insurance.

A case can still be made, though, for having individuals pay only premiums equal to the expected losses they face. The case can be made by either moral or economic efficiency arguments. The moral argument claims that there is no obligation of justice short of contract between actual individuals; obligations never arise out of fate alone. The intuition behind this view is that if one person is struck by lightning, say, through no act or oversight or inaction of a second person, why should the second person be obligated to help the first one? The first one is not worse off because of the second; the second is not better off because of the first. The reply to this in turn, though, is equally intuitive and stubborn, reflecting a completely different conception of justice. If there is no relevant difference between the two parties (i.e., if the second person is no more deserving than the first), why shouldn't the second person be obligated to share the first's most unfortunate, life-agenda-setting burdens? The whole business of living, after all, is a gratuitous fortune for each person, so the pooling of undeserved burdens is part of the very bargain of life. Obligations simply are not grounded only in contract. Thus, if competitive insurers segment the market according to likelihoods of illness, that is simply reason to say that competitive delivery systems are fundamentally flawed.

For most, I suspect, this defense of pooling burdens is persuasive. There is a more telling argument for segmenting premiums, though: efficiency. If everyone pays at the same common community rate, then since less healthy clients do not pay their own way, insurers will try to avoid insuring them. If insurers successfully avoid them, these higher-risk individuals will be left even worse off than they would be with higher premiums but at least insurance, so we will have to compel insurers to accept all applicants. But then high-risk individuals will buy too much coverage—inefficiently much. They will flock to such community-rated insurance—to them it is underpriced. Worse yet, low-risk persons will buy inefficiently little insurance, some of them even going without it altogether because the only coverage they can get seems overpriced. This will happen no matter how stringently community rating is enforced.

There is a more efficient way to accomplish the goal of not leaving the likely ill with greater expense than mandating common premiums: we could allow segmented premiums but then use an explicit, tax-financed subsidy to compensate certifiably less healthy people for their higher costs. People would be eligible for the subsidy on roughly the same grounds used by insurance companies to put people in higher premium brackets (exceptions might be conditions the society regards as distinctly controllable, e.g., smoking).[19]

This argument against mandated community rating might be persuasive, but there is still the further issue of adverse selection. Suppose that, for efficiency or whatever other reason, we allow differentiated premiums. The more expensive plans cover more things with less cost sharing, appealing thereby to a more likely ill clientele. Insurers set rates for such plans accordingly, but they cannot detect the higher-risk status of some who will subscribe (who perhaps can sense their own health status better than any physician or insurance company). In the long run such adverse selection is death to an insurer in a competitive market, who gets stuck with extra losses and then by experience has to raise premiums even higher for this fuller coverage, driving away some of the less likely ill who initially subscribed. But such adverse selection by subscribers leads insurers to respond in kind. They will develop a clever tactic of their own—cream skimming—designing particular coverages to pick off lower risks than the competition attracts with its own packages. Is there anything wrong with an insurance company doing this?

To give a decent assessment of cream skimming we need to go back to adverse selection. On the face of it there is nothing wrong at all with insurers' attempts to avoid adverse selection. Why should a particular plan's subscribers have to pay more to support the likely ill than other subscribers in society have to pay? If a plan does not defend itself against adverse selection, it will find itself doing just that; it has little reason to think other people will carry their share.[20] Just avoiding adverse selection, however, is not where this insurance company behavior is likely to stop. Some insurers will positively try to attract a healthier than average clientele with their own coverages. But generally, if an insurer thus skims cream in some dimension of its coverage, it loses the argument against the legitimacy of adverse selection in other areas. If a plan is skimming cream in one place, then, to be fair to the ill, why should it not carry some of the burden of adverse selection elsewhere?

Yet here, too, there are complexities. Some reasons of fairness support insurers in their efforts to avoid adverse selection and may even support them in trying to attract healthier subscribers with lower premiums.

The most obvious reason here concerns voluntary life-styles. Some needs for care are created by people's individually controllable behaviors, though which needs and behaviors these are in particular cases is notoriously difficult to determine. Most tend to think it fair, for example, to charge smokers higher annual premiums; that is not considered unfair cream skimming or avoidance of adverse selection. There is, however, a well-known problem here. It then seems unfair not also to charge more for overeaters or for hypertensives who do little to control their stress.

In all these cases, the correct standard probably lies along the following lines. A category of subscribers may be asked to constitute its own pool and pay more for its care if (and only if) (1) their cost-creating behavior is accurately detectable (few false negatives and especially few false positives), (2) their behavior is largely voluntary (if not immediately voluntary, then voluntary in that they can take critical steps somewhere else in the background of their lives), and (3) discouraging this behavior does not encroach on fundamentally important areas of personal freedom.

This is only a rough and preliminary discussion of a complicated and highly charged issue, and I have not provided here any kind of careful defense of these three criteria.[21] But suppose that somethng like them is correct. While competitive parties will certainly try to step outside these lines in devising their coverages, competitive systems might be controlled by these moral guidelines if the community has a sufficiently clear sense of them. At any rate, governmentally funded delivery systems will confront many of the same essential controversies in their own parallel taxation policies, which can range from discriminatory to sensible in taxing unhealthy life-styles. If moral criteria are important in that government taxation context, why should they not be equally important for a competitive system that is allowed to serve the public? Either providers and insurers will have to translate the moral sense about these matters into private regulation of their own behavior, or the society will have to step in with supplementary legislation.

In many cases beyond voluntary life-styles it will also be difficult to tell the difference between objectionable cream skimming and legitimate attempts to avoid adverse selection. Suppose a plan decides to put more resources into better prevention and less into remedial treatment (say, heart and liver transplants, to draw a particularly dramatic contrast). Does that plan legitimately avoid the adverse selection of a higher than average number of potential heart and liver failure patients, or does it objectionably skim the cream of subscribers least worried about their hearts and livers? One of the first considerations might appear to be whether other insurers are covering such transplants, but not even that can give us the final answer. Suppose most other plans in the region do cover these transplants but that few offer as well-integrated preventive services as the plan being judged. Would it be wrong in deciding not to cover the transplants and instead upgrade what its members judge to be, dollar for dollar, more beneficial preventive programs?[22]

I think the answer in such a case is perfectly clear. If this plan's emphasis on prevention and not covering some expensive remedial services reflects the genuine beliefs and values of its members about what is the best overall balance of medicine, and if those who opt for other insurers just differ from them in those values and beliefs, then how can anyone, even people most likely to need these procedures, plausibly object to this group's decision not to cover heart and liver transplants as cream skimming?[23] The difficulty, of course, in the actual frenzy of real competition, is distinguishing what is legitimate reflection of honestly various values and beliefs and what is calculated cream skimming. Perhaps we should continue to have our doubts here about what is which—uncertainty will properly keep us on our toes.

Patient cost sharing is another difficult case in which to decide whether what we are facing is objectionable cream skimming. Amid competition, cost-sharing policies will enjoy a certain popularity. While 30 percent of employers included deductibles or copayments for hospital stays in their health insurance plans in 1982, 63 percent had included them by 1985. Some companies are also adopting individual reserve funds which essentially constitute cost sharing, though they may not appear so. ALCOA, for example, deposits $700 in an individual account for each employee; the portion of that account not used for health-care charges during the year reverts to the employee as cash.[24]

The main argument for cost sharing is straightforward efficiency. Giving patients an immediate incentive not to make unnecessary use of medical services reduces total monies spent on health care. That may reduce premiums enough to make it worth consumers' while to give up the financial and security advantages of first-dollar, no-copayment coverage. Especially if stop-loss provisions are used to limit their financial liability for catastrophic care, cost-sharing packages will often be beneficial to thoughtful consumers. Cost sharing's problem, though, is the same general interpersonal problem of equity seen in other cases of possible cream skimming: these arrangements will be much more attractive to the likely well than to the likely ill. Are they wrongly so? On the one hand, people put legitimately different values on the financial security and extra predictability of care that full coverage buys. On the other hand, probably the most common reason people pick a cheaper plan with cost sharing is simply financial: will they end up paying more or not? As in most real cases we have here a mixture of different motivations and effects, and it is very difficult to come to an overall evaluation.

There is another, more definitive problem with cost sharing, however: equity not between well and ill but between rich and poor. Cost-sharing arrangements are much more likely to attract higher-income consumers than relatively poor ones no matter how distinct their cost-containment success might be.

I do not have in mind here the problem that deductibles and copayments hit lower-income families much harder in the real human pocketbook than they hit wealthier ones. That problem can be rectified by graduating any cost-sharing provisions with income.[25] The problem is more fundamental. Of all parties, lower-income families put the highest value on avoiding unforeseen financial contingencies. From a really wide range of options, would the poor in their own self-interest choose a plan with cost sharing? Even if cost sharing discourages much more marginal than basic care, to the relatively poor it is probably still one of the worst ways of doing that. While a narrower range of health care is worth its price to the poor compared to the rich, the poor are more likely to find insuring for whatever care is costworthy a much better buy than will the rich. The poor will likely find lean plans without cost sharing an even better buy than lean plans with it. Knowledgeable lower-income consumers will err on the side of secure financial coverage even if that means a plan that provides fewer marginal services. They are not likely to accept cost sharing in exchange for a wider range of services. This carries an extremely important lesson: if providers are serious about matching their product with the real needs of lower-income clients, they will have to learn to ration care instead of using cost sharing to shift the responsibility for those hard immediate decisions to individual patients.[26]

Does all of this mean that it is unfair both to the likely ill and to the relatively poor to have cost-sharing plans in the marketplace? Perhaps, but not necessarily. Employee groups marked by wide variation in income and likelihood of illness need to be very careful not to embrace cost-sharing arrangements just because they are good bargains for the average employee. They might not be a good bargain at all either to those on the low end of the company's pay scale or to those who expect to incur major medical expenses. This does not mean that employers should not offer cost-sharing options; it just requires employers to include one or more first-dollar coverage options that are no more expensive than the cost-sharing arrangements. If in fact providers and insurers are not offering any such equally inexpensive full-coverage option, then, yes, something is wrong with cost sharing. But it would still not be clear whether that was the fault of a highly competitive insurance market itself. It could be, for example, that providers are stubborn in refusing to do the required rationing, thus limiting what insurers can realistically offer.

Note, too, that reservations about cost sharing are no final reason to prefer government regulation over market competition as a strategy for containing costs. The cost-containment pressures creating cost sharing in a private, competitive economy might also create it in a more government-dominated arrangement. The only systems likely to avoid more of the cost sharing that is objectionable to the poor and the ill than competition are a truly nationalized health service or a relatively noncompetitive, unregulated medical economy. Those options raise other problems, so it is much too simple just to reject competition because it leads to inequitable cost sharing.

From all these points we can grope toward a complex conclusion. What may look like cream skimming or morally mindless scrambling to avoid adverse selection is not always objectionable. Certainly, however, there is in competition a very significant danger of discrimination against the likely ill. Community rating as a direction for policy is inefficient, but if we do not mandate it, we will have to subsidize the discernibly likely ill for their higher premiums. Anyone urging competition as an arrangement for health-care delivery should realize how careful we must be about all of this.[27]

Telling Patients about Care Withheld

In competition some plans and providers will not be offering all the care that might benefit a particular patient regardless of its cost. One of its major goals as health-care policy is to force consumers and thereby insurers and providers to make serious decisions about whether marginal units of care are worth what they cost. Some subscribers will consent to take the necessary risk of prospectively forgoing certain beneficial care if they thereby save enough to use for other things. Rationing care is permitted—nay, demanded—by consumers' prior consent when they knowledgeably pick cheaper, leaner plans.

But while rationing is thus justified in outline, how in particular are physicians and other providers to behave toward patients? One question here is whether they ought to become active rationing agents. Over time competitive frameworks will create tremendous pressures for providers to do that, and some arguments support it as well. How can the best decisions on these matters possibly be made by regulation from up top, with little discretion from individual clinicians?[28] Suppose, then that providers become partially active rationing agents.

Of course, plans should still get as much up-front consumer input as possible on what to ration. That can be done through member involvement in a plan's actual policymaking or by the disbursement of good information to present and prospective subscribers about the rationing policies and decisions actually used. But if there is neither appreciable consumer governance nor sufficient subscriber information, much of the prior consent justification for rationing polices gets lost. At least what is then left of the justification of rationing is at odds with respect for the autonomy and dignity of consumers and patients.[29]

Now assume that all of this has been considered. Consumers are either directly making a plan's rationing policies or being adequately informed about them. Physicians and other providers are still, however, using their discretion in individually rationing care when no sufficiently detailed policy instructs them in what to do. We come to the further question I want to take up in this section: when a particular provider then properly uses his or her discretion and decides not to prescribe some specific potentially beneficial piece of care because it appears to cost too much for its likely benefits, should the provider inform the patient that he or she has done precisely that? We already know in which direction competitive pressures will lie: not to inform patients for fear they will leave for other plans.[30]

There is at least one respectable argument for not having to tell, and that is if the information would not be material to the patient. Imagine a parallel situation in Britain. A patient older than sixty-five is not going to be prescribed dialysis though it could do him some good. His internist does not think he is a sufficiently outstanding exception to the general rule that dialysis is too expensive for that category of patient. Should the internist describe for him the situation and decision, in effect bringing him into the discussion of his own rationing case? One observer finds it "difficult to imagine any discussion a patient would find more stressful. Desperate, arguing for life . . . , the patient may find himself denuded of privacy and self-respect."[31] And to virtually no effect. The patient has little recourse—the information is not "material" to anything he can do to get the treatment he is denied. In a competitive framework, whether the information is material will focus more on ability to switch plans or pay for insurance. "If the patient is unlikely to be able to pay for the treatment" out of pocket after being told it is available but being denied, "might it not then be cruel and pointless to tell him of its existence? Should a Mississippi dirt farmer be told of an expensive cancer treatment available at Sloan-Kettering that has a one in a thousand chance of saving his life . . . ?[32]

In part we have to agree. If the care in question is not even close to what such a patient would choose to have included in a plan that he or she would purchase with available resources, then informing the patient is not at all material. Moreover, it is not information that people would want to have if they knew they could get it.[33] Here is the most important consideration: *if the information really could realistically lead the patient to make some other decision,* like purchasing the care out of pocket, or joining another plan whose providers could be known to ration things differently for a price also within reach of the patient, *then the provider is obligated to make the information available.*[34]

I can see no way around this conclusion without destroying the entire consent justification for rationing. The resources of the plan are not just the property of the plan, to be meted out to subscribers at its whim as if it were some stockholders' corporation or private foundation deciding how to use its money. The plan's resources are not independently owned by the plan; they are what comes in directly from subscribers' willingness to pay.[35] Prior consent to being in this particular plan is simply impotent as moral support for rationing if the information currently in question might change a person's consent. One can even make a case, parallel to informed consent law, that providers should be legally obligated to provide this information when it is material. And even if it is not material but still the patient would want to have it, the provider ought to inform.

This conclusion is undoubtedly extremely disturbing to providers. They now not only have to act sometimes as rationing agents but in effect they have to tell patients when something statistically beneficial is being withheld, unless that information is neither material nor something patients would want to know.

This might be tempered by other factors in some situations. Compare how the obligation to provide information to dying patients about their terminal condition might arguably be modified. There one does not always need to give the information straight out. One might at first only suggest it, then wait for the patient to respond and ask. Perhaps the same could be done with information about rationing. "Well, there's something that might help, but the odds are awfully slim." That can be an ideal opener to the patient concerned about his or her plan being too restrictive on care. Could it then be argued that if the patient does not inquire further a provider is not obligated to inform him or her more precisely?

I suspect that this way of tempering the general conclusion that providers must tell their patients that care is being rationed is on the right track, but it is certainly treacherous. For one thing, an important informed consent case, *Truman* v. *Thomas,* seems to lean the other way.[36] For years a woman was urged by her physician to get a Pap smear. She consistently refused and then contracted cervical cancer. She died, and her survivors successfully sued the physician for not having directly and more forcefully told her the specific reasons for having the test. The doctor noted that he had urged her to have the test and had even offered to provide it free of charge, and he argued that since she had then never asked for the reasons, he was not obligated to provide them. The court disagreed. The doctor was obligated to provide information as vital as the reasons for Pap smears even if the patient had had ample opportunity to ask and had not. Perhaps this case is relevently different from information about rationing—it involved cancer and its ominous prospects, the Pap smear test was easy and cheap, and so on. But even if we should thus conclude that providers are obligated only to invite their patients to ask about rationing information, we must be very careful that this does not turn into a blanket excuse not to inform.

Furthermore, we have to be very wary of paternalism. Physicians may easily come to believe that for patients' own good they should not be told that possibly beneficial care is being withheld. That is not sufficient reason for not telling, unless we were to countenance paternalistic deception in more traditional situations also. Because of obvious possible conflicts of interest, medical paternalism in the new situation would seem to "take on . . . [an] even more damning kind of odium."[37] "For the patient's own good" will not do. What we must be able to argue is that the patient would really approve of the provider withholding the information if he or she could reflect on this sort of case.

Again we have come face to face with a tremendous moral problem for competition. But here again also, as with cost shifting and cream skimming, the problem's complexity precludes easy dismissal of competitive arrangements as always or finally more objectionable than other structures for delivering medicine. If society continues to pursue competitive approaches, we will have to be more on our moral guard than we have been. Some of the morally mandatory restrictions or supplements, such as adequate public assistance for those who cannot afford to pay and corrective subsidies to the predictably, chronically ill, will require a political will largely missing up to now. Unless insurers, providers, and consumers talk out these problems openly, we will never find competition finally conscionable.

NOTES

1. For discussions of the for-profit issue itself, see Brock and Buchanan (1985) and Veatch (1985).

2. A strong reason for using resources on one good rather than another is simply that the people affected ultimately prefer that good. The "ultimately" qualification is crucial. Of course, people make mistakes about what will satisfy their preferences in the long run. But even then their preferences still finally determine the goals in reference to which the effectiveness of their intermediate decisions and desires is measured.

3. Reimbursement of hospitals by *diagnostic related groups*.

4. Reinhardt (1987), p. 173.

5. Most employer-paid health insurance premiums are currently excluded from taxable income. That is, money channeled to health care through such premiums avoids social security tax (7 percent for both the employer and the employee separately), one's marginal income tax (more than 20 percent on the average), and any state and local income taxes. See Brandon (1982) and Menzel (1983), pp. 127–33.

6. Stein (1985).

7. Ginzberg (1987). For a more specific study comparing hospital charges in competitive versus noncompetitive locales, see Robinson and Luft (1987). For a general skepticism about deregulation, see Kinzer (1988).

8. The need to cover unreimbursed care intensified even before recent DRG policies and the high unemployment and budget cutbacks of the early 1980s. The percentage of hospital

charges not reimbursed by Medicare was already rising—from 14 percent in 1975, for example, to 23 percent in 1981. The likely explanation lies largely in the fact that nonprofit hospitals were increasingly using normal-market, interest-paying methods of obtaining capital as donated capital became scarce. Already in the 1970s Medicare did not include capital expenses in its cost-reimbursement formulas for recoverable charges. See Ginsburg and Sloan (1984), pp. 894–95.

9. Kessel (1958).

10. For a longer explanation of the importance of these distributions of power and resources, see Menzel (1983), pp. 4–15.

11. To the extent that it does not and the revenue comes from charitable donations, competition will not exert pressure against providing unreimbursed care.

12. For arguments for a collective obligation instead of rights to health care, see Buchanan (1984), especially p. 77.

13. See the data collected by Meyer (1983), pp. 10–24, and the revenue option chart in Table 2. The lowest two personal income quintiles in the United States pay exactly the same percentage of the hospital cost shift for unreimbursed care as their respective percentages of total income in the society. The third quintile pays 6 percent more, the fourth 3 percent more, and the top quintile 8 percent less.

14. Mitchell and Vogel (1975) and Brandon (1982).

15. Meyer (1983), pp. 10–24.

16. A politically influential view behind the full current income exclusion is espoused by the United Auto Workers: it is wrong to tax a private substitute for what should be a societal obligation (universal comprehensive health insurance). See Hoffman (1985). As an argument, this is weak. Suppose that provision of comprehensive health insurance is society's obligation. To pay for this insurance the average auto worker's taxes would then be considerably higher than they presently are. The current employer-paid premium, not needing to be used directly to buy insurance, could become part of the worker's income, and then that higher income would be taxed to fund the government insurance. The worker would probably have to be taxed at least as much as if employer-paid premiums were taxed in the current situation.

17. Sager (1988). No one who reads Sager's account, however, will think the political future for such programs easy. Note also that another part of the larger discussion of political feasibility depends on what constitutes minimally decent care. If minimally decent care for the poor can be a noticeably leaner package of care than that which seems decent to most of the middle class, it might be politically easier than most observers think to get the society to guarantee its access. See Chapter 7 for the argument that such a lower level can be acceptable. Note that the argument there even admits that the existing distribution of income is unjust.

18. Pauly (1988), p. 68.

19. The argument in this and the previous paragraph is taken straight from Pauly (1988), pp. 52–53. For an equally lucid and insightful treatment, see Pauly (1984). On further complications, especially in the context of prepaid plans, see Luft (1986).

20. Another reason why it might be fair for a group to avoid adverse selection has emerged from the recent controversies over the practice of age-rating premiums. Suppose that the more likely ill elderly who now pay higher dues previously paid lower premiums when they were in their own younger, cheaper, healthier years. If higher and lower premiums thus balance out over their lifetimes, insurers' use of premium differentials to reduce adverse selection does not seem unfair.

21. For one of the best treatments, see Veatch (1980).

22. A real case in point might be Group Health Cooperative of Puget Sound (GHC), a large prepaid plan in Washington. (See the second section of Chapter 1.) At one point GHC's Heart and Liver Transplant Coverage Subcommittee recommended not covering heart and adult liver transplants, though a new heart transplant center had opened in Seattle and the

majority of carriers in the area by then covered those transplants. If GHC had stuck with that initial recommendation, would it have been objectionably skimming cream? I think not. Some of its reasons for not putting resources into these transplants at that time were the competing needs in prevention and health-promotion programs and in-patient psychiatric services, and the organization had a long-standing commitment to preventive care.

23. One of the few treatments in distributive justice theory that considers the peculiar role of varying beliefs is Yaari and Bar-Hillel (1984), pp. 15–19. For a suggestively related discussion of when people should have to accept certain disadvantages to themselves created by others' religious and moral beliefs, see Calabresi (1985), especially pp. 45–86. It is not clear, though, whether anything can be transferred to health insurance from his discussion of tort liability and constitutional values. If one ignores this problem and just plows ahead, one might draw from Calabresi the following implications. Others should not have to share the extra bill for one's more expensive health care if it results from one's nonreligious, relatively idiosyncratic beliefs and one is in a better position than others to judge what scope of health care is necessary and efficient in protecting one's interests and reflecting one's values. But if the higher bill results form one's religious and relatively common beliefs and others are in at least as good a position to judge the appropriate scope of care, they should have to share in one's higher bill.

24. Stein (1985).

25. Graduating deductibles and copayments has seemed practically difficult to many observers. In fact it is probably completely feasible with new computer facilities. Xerox Corporation, for example, makes an individual employee's annual deductible simply 1 percent of his or her annual pay, with a stop-loss on the subsequent 20 percent copayment of 4 percent of annual pay. Stein (1985).

26. A somewhat different version of this argument appears in Menzel (1983), pp. 122–23.

27. One of the main proponents of competitive strategies, Alain Enthoven, has made many concrete suggestions about how to guard against unfairly high premiums for the ill. See Enthoven (1978). For specific suggestions, see also Butler (1980) and Menzel (1983), p. 141.

28. See Chapter 1.

29. The consent can be presumed, but only if there are very good reasons for bypassing actual consent that are themselves morally faithful to consumers; see Chapter 2. For many other points in favor of making rationing policies public, see Winslow (1986).

30. It is not impossible for competitive forces to work in the other direction. A plan might get an extremely trusted reputation over a long period of time because, among other things, it keeps its patients in the know on such matters as this.

31. Halper (1985), p. 81.

32. Baily (1986), p. 20.

33. The idea here is the same as the "material information" standard of informed consent law—information that might actually lead the patient to make a different decision. See *Cobbs* v. *Grant,* 502 P. 2d 1 (1972). The "want to know" standard is more demanding (most people want to have a considerable amount of information that does not lead to any new decisions). The argument that what one wants to know is the proper moral standard, regardless of its legal status, is simply that people's thoughts and desires and not just their decisions and behavior are very important to them.

34. Mehlman (1986), p. 861, suggests a similar standard.

35. This is the defect of the "private property" objection to morally required publicity made by D. Friedman (1986), pp. 218–19.

36. *Truman* v. *Thomas,* 611 P. 2d 902 (1980).

37. Stone (1985), p. 312, speaking, though, about the witholding of the care itself, not the withholding of the information about it that is the focus here.

9

Malpractice and the Costs of Complaint

Suppose we endorse restraining health care according to its costs and benefits. Providers take account of the resources they use, not just the individual medical needs of their patients. Ideally, decisions to forgo possibly beneficial care are based on patients' actual prior consent, but where that is not feasible providers act according to policies patients would have presumably accepted. Currently uninsured segments of the population are covered by an expanded Medicaid program. There, in Medicare, and in private insurance, devices such as DRGs (payment by diagnostic related group) turn on the heat of competition. The restrained care that results still reflects commitment to individuals as real persons—people living consciously over time, trying to be careful of their own resources, caring at least minimally about the larger society in which they live.[1]

If such a view of disciplined medicine is propounded to providers they will immediately note the threat of malpractice suits, which they feel would undo the whole lot of such well-intentioned restraints. Medical liability suits have grown in recent years—in number, in the size of awards, and in the conceptual scope of the protections they afford to patients. How, then, can hospitals, nurses, and doctors be expected to forgo any significant number of procedures just because that saves resources better used elsewhere? When they get sued for not having done more, do we really expect them to use as their courtroom defense the expense of the treatment they passed over?

As astonishing as it may seem, I think we can expect providers to defend themselves that way. Defensive medicine is a significant factor in rising health-care costs, but a qualified, consent-based defense of expense can be made—and as not only an academic but a real legal argument. A major barrier to using such an argument is the mistaken belief that a more general, apparently similar defense in tort law, a plaintiff's assumption of risk, is now virtually dead. To the contrary, I will argue that insofar as general assumption of risk is similar to a consent-based defense of expense, assumption of risk is not hopelessly outmoded at all. Furthermore, providers need not fear any no-fault liability when medical restraint sometimes leaves unfortunate victims.

Defensive Medicine

Liability suits have undoubtedly constituted a cost-escalating pressure in medicine. In the state of Washington, for example, a physician's average annual malpractice insurance premium in 1986 topped $15,000; nationally the average premium rose at an annual rate of 21.4 percent from 1982 to 1985. Nationally before 1978, an average of 3.3 claims a year were filed against every 100 physicians; between 1980 and 1983, 7.8 a year; in 1983, 9.3. A median jury verdict was already $200,000 by 1982; for infant plaintiffs, it was $1.4 million. By 1984, judgments for plaintiffs of all ages, including out-of-court settlements, averaged more than $300,000.[2]

The American Medical Association estimated in 1984 that malpractice insurance premiums added $5 to the cost of an office visit and $15 to a hospital day.[3] Accounting for other significant categories of expense makes the full costs of liability suits much larger yet:

1. Provider's premiums ($8 billion to $12 billion range)	$10 billion[4]
2. Drug manufacturers' premiums	2 billion
3. Defensive medicine ($10 billion to $52 billion range)	30 billion
Total cost increase ($20 billion to $66 billion range)	42 billion
Of this, total awarded to plaintiffs	5 billion[5]
Apparent net loss	37 billion

There is much room for variance in estimating some of these components. The main point of dispute is defensive medicine, the added cost from services provided in reaction to the threat of suit. The AMA claims that $52 billion per year is spent on such defensive medicine, and a recent related analysis puts the bill for defensive physician services alone at $10.6 billion for 1984.[6] Competing analyses, however, put the total costs of defensive medicine much lower than $52 billion.

The key to understanding the lower estimates is to note carefully the definition of *defensive medicine:* improper care prescribed because of the threat of suit.[7] Defensive medicine in an economically interesting sense is not just all care caused by the perceived threat of suit. It is only poor, unjustified care so caused. Also, much of what passes for defensive medicine might actually be caused by other factors: incentives for services created by insurance, fee-for-service reimbursement, or the nature of physician's medical education, to name just a few.[8]

So there is a hidden saving in malpractice liability: the threat of suit may deter considerable amounts of unjustified practice that would lead to greater detriment than that caused by defensive medicine. Patricia Danzon, perhaps the foremost economist in this area, calculates this benefit to patients who would otherwise have been victims of shoddy practice at $10 billion.[9] Added to the $5 billion legally awarded to actual victims and with defensive medicine's real cost at $10 billion, not $52 billion, her estimate of the total net cost of malpractice liability looks much different from the AMA's:

1. Providers' insurance premium $10 billion
2. Drug manufacturer's premiums   2 billion
3. Defensive medicine   10 billion

   Total cost increase   22 billion
   Benefit to actual and potential victims 15 billion
   Apparent net loss   7 billion

Even here, however, the institution of malpractice liability has a significant net cost. We could even make the net cost zero if we could just cut defensive medicine by two-thirds. This should demonstrate that while the problem of defensive medicine can be easily overblown, it should concern anyone who wants resources used wisely. Particularly if the personal costs of prospectively being sued loom large in provider's minds, malpractice suits will be a major barrier to their ever internalizing an ethic of efficiently rationing care. Tort law must come to grips with this. Practitioners should not look slavishly to tort law for their morality. It should work the other way around: tort law should be determined by the most considered view of providers' moral obligations to their patients.

A Consent-Based Defense of Expense

The basic concern about medical malpractice is certainly not to minimize malpractice awards; to effectively encourage proper practice, in fact, maybe total awards should be even higher than they are. The basic concern is instead a moral one: in what circumstances should a consumer of health care be com-

pensated for gambles that go awry? A practitioner goes short on some particular item of care because of its expense, and an unlucky patient ends up dead
or damaged—call that the injury, though it happened by omission.[10] Should
the patient be compensated for it? Suppose the patient is one of the few, it
turns out, whom the extra bit of care would have saved.

In forming impressions about where the law might come down in such
medical cases we must be careful not to misinterpret some famous cases in
other areas of tort law where the preservation of life apparently assumed an
overriding importance. For example, in 1871, a man named Eckert daringly
rushed to save a little girl playing on the tracks of the Long Island Railroad
oblivious to an oncoming train. Apparently he had little chance of saving her,
and even then not without great risk to himself. As it turned out, she lived
and he was killed. His survivors sued the railroad, arguing that the railroad
negligently failed to protect against trespassers. The railroad did not deny this
but claimed that Eckert had contributed his own negligence, dashing to save
the child with such a high risk to himself and small chance of saving her. The
court resoundingly rejected the railroad's claim: "The law has so high a regard
for human life that it will not impute negligence to an effort to preserve it."
Maybe Eckert's heroism was foolish, but he was clean in the eyes of the law.[11]

The law veritably oozes here with reverence for vulnerable, innocent life
and the heroic effort to save it, yet the decision sets no precedent whatsoever
for the current question of whether doctors and nurses are liable if they decide
not to pull out every stop in their medical arsenal. *Eckert* does tell us something about a provider's liability if he or she goes beyond the call of duty (in
Good Samaritan rescue situations, for example), but it tells us nothing about
where the line of duty itself should be seen to fall. That, however, is the issue
in the defense of expense.

Let's stand back for a minute to get the larger picture. People usually think
that tort law should accomplish two goals: to see that the defendant and the
plaintiff get what they deserve and to encourage their optimal behavior. On
the defendant's desert, we lean toward a negligence requirement. The plaintiff
must show that the defendant has been negligent, but the defendant can dilute
this by showing that the plaintiff contributed his or her own negligence.[12] On
what the plaintiff deserves, we are often torn. The plaintiff clearly deserves an
award when he or she has been wronged by a negligent defendant, but we may
think he or she deserves something even when the defendant has not been
negligent. Suppose that the plaintiff's unlucky plight is not in any sense the
defendant's fault, but the defendant is well positioned to pass on the costs of
any judgment to a wider pool of patients who benefit from his or her practice.
We will then be inclined toward strict liability—holding the defendant liable
for compensation to the plaintiff even when no one has been negligent.[13]

The other goal, encouraging optimal behavior by both defendant and plaintiff, comes in at the more fundamental level of setting the standard of negligent behavior itself. An important consideration is efficiency. We do not want people chasing too small or improbable a catch with too expensive a lure, but on the other hand we do not want them passing up bait that is likely to catch more than it costs. Outside the area of medical malpractice, the use of economic efficiency to determine standards of liability has a distinguished history.[14] Cases involving economic efficiency in medical liability, however, are rare. To make matters worse for anyone proposing a defense of expense, one of them, *Helling* v. *Carey,* has widened, not narrowed, physician liability.[15] On several counts, however, *Helling* still provides a perfect entrance into our discussion.

Thirty-two-year-old Mrs. Helling sued Dr. Carey for her blindness from glaucoma. Carey would have detected the glaucoma and prevented the blindness had he performed a simple five-dollar test, tonometry. At the time the standard of the profession was not to perform it routinely on patients younger than forty; for one thing, the incidence of glaucoma then is very small, one in 25,000. Carey cited this custom of his profession and might have said, "Even if my profession is wrong, why should *I* have to pay for Mrs. Helling's misfortune? You can't even say I should have known better."

The Washington State Supreme Court was hardly fazed by the argument. It told him in effect, "It makes no difference that we shouldn't blame you as an individual physician. We really shouldn't, but we will hold you liable nonetheless. That will keep your profession on its toes, and anyway, you will be able to spread the cost of any such judgment out among all your other patients. That will be fairer than simply leaving blind Mrs. Helling uncompensated."

Then the court got to the primary question, undistracted by concerns about individual blame. Is the routine omission of tonometry for patients younger than forty justifiable medical practice? To the court its decision here did not seem terribly difficult. In part it applied the famous Hand efficiency test for reasonable care: negligence occurs when it costs less to prevent a mishap than to pay for the damages predicted to result from it.[16] More formally:

Negligence: Cost of Prevention (CP) is less than Accident Loss
            discounted by Accident Probability (AP)
      N: $CP < (AL \times AP)$

In *Helling* v. *Carey* in particular:

$CP = \$5$
$AL = \$678,000$[17]

AP = 1/25,000

Test: Is $5 < (\$678,000 \times 1/25,000)$?
Yes: $5 < \$27$
Thus: Dr. Carey is negligent

Some will object that this is an incredibly arbitrary calculation. In this analysis $678,000 is the actual average jury award for blindness from 1973 to 1977 (the relevant period of the lawsuit). How can we be remotely confident that this represents the monetary value people place on their sight? Suppose that other factors than the value of sight alone are wittingly or unwittingly included in such jury awards, so we reduce $678,000 to $500,000.[18] Most people are also risk-averse,[19] so the value of eliminating the 1-in-25,000 risk of blindness accomplished by the tonometry is more than just the straight accident loss discounted by the risk; probably, however, juries have already determined their awards for blindness with that in mind. Juries also probably think of how far off the normal scale of good and bad the prospect of being blind is compared to the things we usually buy with money, so they quite properly award on the high side of any particular money figure they can see as a substitute for the value of sight. If all that is correct, then somewhere between twenty dollars and thirty dollars is the right break-even point for determining negligence after all. That is hardly a precise estimate, but it can still be helpful in practice. Using the actual five-dollar tonometry test, if that is all it really costs, is clearly efficient, while using a fifty-dollar one would clearly not be.

We talk about this argument in terms of just efficiency, but morally it amounts to much more than that. People's own consent is right at the heart of the matter. Clear-headed people who value sight in the half-million-dollar range would not just think that such a five-dollar test should be used in a plan to which they were contributing—they would demand that it be used. The five-dollar test falls below the twenty- to thirty-dollar break point by such a large margin that it becomes entirely safe to presume that people would pay the increased premium to fund such tests. On the facts about tonometry and glaucoma as they were taken to be in this case, it would have been insulting to patients if the court had not reversed professional custom.

We should not make the mistake of thinking that since *Helling* held the doctor liable the case portends wider overall liability for providers. The reasoning of this case may actually reduce providers' liability in the long run. In *Helling,* suppose that because of indirect hidden costs, the real expense of tonometry was fifty dollars, not five dollars. Then the Hand formula would require the conclusion that the physician was not negligent:

Negligence: $CP < (AL \times AP)$
   Test: Is $\$50 < (\$678{,}000 \times 1/25{,}000)$?
    No: $\$50 > \$27$
   Thus: The doctor is not negligent

The court would have had to clear Carey of charges of negligence in omitting tonometry for Mrs. Helling. The custom of not using tonometry for normal patients younger than forty would have been efficient, and it would have accorded with our best guess of the policy to which people would have consented beforehand.

Some commentators on *Helling,* indeed, have argued that a set of facts precisely like these is closer to the truth about tonometry than the five-dollar figure on which the court seemed to make its decision. Fortess and Kapp claim that the large number of false positives turned up by routine use of the test will need to be followed up, creating enormous expense beyond the modest five-dollar cost of the initial test itself.[20] The real cost per initial test turns out to be more than fifty dollars.

Nothing of particular interest would have been raised in the real *Helling* case if the court at the time had thought that the costs of tonometry were actually this high; lacking any economic ammunition with which to challenge the custom of the profession, the plaintiff would have lost. But now, later, after accommodating ourselves to the real *Helling* decision as we have, learning that the total cost of tonometry exceeds fifty dollars creates the prospect of an exceptionally interesting suit. It is now the custom of the profession to administer tonometry routinely to people younger than forty, at least in states such as Washington governed by *Helling.* Suppose a doctor and his colleagues read Fortess and Kapp and suspect that tonometry's hidden costs make it inefficient for normal patients younger than forty. They carefully study the matter further, conclude that indeed the per test real costs are up at least around fifty dollars, and abandon routine use on clients younger than forty. As a result, one of their patients goes blind. She sues. The doctor acknowledges the general practice of routine tonometry but defends himself by noting that the real cost per test is way above the twenty- to thirty-dollar break-even efficiency range, say fifty dollars.

Why shouldn't the doctor win? The key moral point in the actual *Helling* decision is that people would demand inclusion of a five-dollar tonometry test to prevent one case of blindness every 25,000 tries. The point in our new hypothetical case is parallel: it is virtually as clear that people would consent to exclude a fifty-dollar test.

No one can say, of course, that if this case were real the doctor would actually win in court. Fortess and Kapp correctly note, for one thing, how few jurisdictions have followed *Helling* in overturning a customary standard of the profession.[21] Several factors, however, greatly increase the chances that a court will enforce or allow behavior at variance with typical professional practice. Perhaps most important is the ability to cite a recognizable minority viewpoint in the professional literature or practice.[22] Note what that practically means in the coming decades: as cost-conscious scholars and practitioners infuse more and more economic accountability into their discussions and clinical recommendations, the defense of expense will naturally become more and more legitimate even if it does not determine the predominant practice pattern.[23]

A defendant provider's particular practice setting may also make a considerable difference. The more clearly and explicitly the entire context is lean delivery and concern about efficiency rather than a no-holds-barred approach of doing everything possible, the more confidently courts can guess that plaintiffs would have consented beforehand to policies forgoing particular procedures. It is also very important to be acting in good faith toward one's patients. If the paramount reason for passing up some item of care seems to be saving money divorced from a consistent, general attempt to offer the best combination of quality and price to one's clientele, then one will be vulnerable to suits of bad faith.[24]

Once efficient rationing becomes an important concern in the culture and health care generally, the case for allowing a qualified, consent-based legal defense of expense becomes compelling. This should be no surprise. Most malpractice suits have assumed that a provider's undivided loyalty ought to be to patients' individual best interests. If moral understanding of loyalty to patients is broadened to take account of their presumable prior consent, both the profession's ethic and legal rulings will have to change.

Assumption of Risk

So there is no lack of good argument for a defense of expense. Why, then, are so many still skeptical that it could ever see the light of day in court? Any full explanation will have to refer to a widespread misimpression people have about an important chapter in tort law history: the assumption of risk defense. It is often thought that this defense is a thing of the past and that its death dooms from the start any defense of expense resting on the similar idea of presumable consent to risk. I will argue that this whole perception of the traditional defense and its import for medical liability is mistaken. We now recognize some uses of assumption of risk to be the moral travesties they were, but though time has shown it to be limited, it is far from dead. Once understood, its limitations are in fact tailor-made for a properly conceived defense of expense.

The key is to understand what has been all along the central limitation of any assumption of risk defense. Suppose we are confident that the plaintiff voluntarily assumed the risk of the harm that has now led him or her to sue the defendants. We should certainly not absolve the defendants if they unreasonably or negligently created or exacerbated that risk. Defendants' duty is defined in relation to the creation of the danger itself. They do not fulfill it merely by warning the prospective plaintiff about a risk he or she then consents to take if it is they who were negligent in contributing to the risk in the first place.[25]

This principle can be ironically illustrated by a famous case in which the plaintiff actually lost. In 1900 an employee, Lamson, complained to American Ax and Tool Company about the newly installed racks on which freshly painted hatchets were hung to dry. He claimed the hatchets could more easily slip from their pegs. The company met his objection bruskly: he was told that those were the new racks, they would stay, and he could either work or leave. The accident he feared soon happened—to him. He sued and lost. The court's decision was stark: "The plaintiff . . . perfectly understood what was likely to happen. That likelihood did not depend upon the doing of some negligent act [by the company] but solely on the permanent conditions of the racks and their surroundings."[26]

Today hardly anyone would agree with that decision against the employee. This even tempts us to abandon the assumption of risk defense. But in fact the principle that the court used is not off base at all. If the company's behavior in installing and not removing the new racks with whatever risks they posed was not negligent, then the company should not be held liable (though if the company's behavior was negligent, then it should be). If today we disagree with the court's decision, it is because we hold a different view of the contingency. We think the company was negligent in installing the new racks to begin with, given the danger they posed, or at least that it was negligent in not modifying or replacing them after Lamson complained.[27]

The same principle is illustrated by many other cases. In *Brown* v. *San Francisco Ball Club* (1950), a spectator was injured by a foul ball while sitting in an unscreened seating area. The court sided with the club, noting that most of the seats were unscreened. The decision against Brown, the court made clear, "does not mean that he assumes the risk of being injured by the proprietor's negligence but [only] that by voluntarily entering into the sport as a spectator he knowingly accepts the *reasonable* risks and hazards inherent in and incident to the game."[28] This principle is also applicable in motorcycle helmet cases. Though a motorcyclist assumes a higher risk of injury by wearing no helmet, another motorist is not absolved from liability if he or she negligently causes the accident.[29] Or if a pedestrian tries to cross a busy street and gets injured, we do not necessarily say, "You knew the risks, so tough luck." The pedestrian may have knowingly and freely decided to cross, but we keep the pressure on the motorist nonetheless. If the motorist was at fault, the plaintiff has a right to damages; if the motorist was not, the pedestrian does not.[30]

I have so far passed over another obvious doubt in cases such as *Lamson*—about his freedom to leave. The issue will turn on duress and coercion, notoriously difficult notions to define. The most persuasive moral and legal analysis of duress, I suspect, requires a coercing party to have violated the risk taker's rights already in setting up the distasteful alternatives among which he or she then has to choose. The proverbial "your money or your life" gunman has clearly done that; a low-wage worker's "clean" employer generally has not.[31] Whether Lamson is acting voluntarily or under duress depends on whether American Ax and Tool has violated Lamson's rights in putting him in his current bind. That in turn simply returns us to whether the company was negligent.

In all these respects the focus stays riveted on the defendant's own negligence. At this point, in turn, the law may resort to economic considerations. The Hand formula encountered in *Helling* can enter, defining negligence as a function of the relative costs of accidents and their prevention. We are comfortable with this, however, only so long as nothing approaching "butchery" is involved—that is, we are comfortable with it only where we have no solid convictions independent of economic factors about the standard of care to which the defendant should be held. Moreover, second-order economic considerations may make it more difficult for defendants to get off the hook with economic reasons than at first we might suppose. Even when a provider's restrained approach to care seems to be efficient in the long run, we might still find him or her negligent for a more subtle reason: the provider might be better situated to assess the risks and determine whether they are worth taking. That may actually have happened in *Lamson;* the court felt very unsure deciding that American Ax's new racks were not fully efficient compared to the previous ones, thinking that Lamson himself was in the best position to judge that whole business. In a modern manufacturing context we might feel quite the opposite—that the company is generally in the better position to judge.[32]

Since the defendant's negligence is still the key issue even when assumption of risk seems to turn our focus to the plaintiff, some legal scholars conclude that assumption of risk is not a real defense at all. In a genuine defense, one would first acknowledge the initial case for liability and then say, "But look, here's the reason I should nevertheless not lose." Assumption of risk does not appear to work that way.

1. When the plaintiff's assumption of risk is *unreasonable,* a real defense is created despite the defendant's admitted negligence, but it is the defense of contributory negligence, not assumption of risk.
2. When the plaintiff's assumption of risk is reasonable but the defendant had a duty not to create or impose that risk (or at least not to impose it in the way he or she did, say with only the warning he or she gave), then the plaintiff's assumption of risk does not protect the defendant.
3. When the plaintiff's assumption of risk is reasonable and the defendant was not negligent in creating or imposing the risk in the first place, the defendant has not breached any duty to the plaintiff; no defense is needed.[33]

All of this helps to clarify the structural place of consent to economic efficiency in medical malpractice law. The legal defense of expense will not focus directly on risks that the plaintiff has assumed. The argument is directly and primarily about whether a provider was negligent. Establishing that the patient assumed a certain risk gives providers no protection whatsoever when they are themselves already negligent, and if they are not negligent, their legal argument will not even need to put forth an official defense.

The importance of an earlier point now becomes much clearer. To use a consent-based defense of expense, a defendant can be at most only very ambiguously negligent. The case must either be one in which the provider is just not negligent or one in which the negligence is clearly open to debate and begs for some additional reasoning such as economic efficiency and consent for resolution. To settle the central moral and legal issue of the provider's negligence, we may admittedly have to refer back to some presumable consent of prospective patients. We did that, for example, in both contrasting versions of the *Helling* case. But doing that is not using assumption of risk directly as a defense; it is only pursuing the necessary moral substance of the negligence issue itself.

In looking toward consent to risk to address the substance of a provider's negligence, of course, subtle options are open to us. We might choose to say that health-care professionals have the duty to provide care regardless of expense unless they can cite some sort of patient/person consent to passing it by. Or we might say they have a duty to provide care only when the client has some background expectation that the care will be given. Undoubtedly there are other ways to shave the substantive duty here into which the consent element fits. It is in some such evolving moral predilections of the society about consent itself that courts will find a necessary part of the material from which to shape an answer to the central question of medical defendants' negligence.

Assumption of risk might, of course, more directly determine a provider's negligence through private contractual arrangements. Some advocates of consumer sovereignty, in fact, have proposed abandoning all tort law standards in favor of individual and group contracts about standards of care.[34] Tort law is inherently coercive, they argue, binding people to the same standard of care regardless of their often legitimately different views. Yet any proposal to substitute explicit contract for the whole of medical malpractice law would confront virtually insuperable problems about sufficiently informing all the contracting parties.[35]

The better approach is to keep tort law but see it as a shelter of background standards hewn by presumptions about the policies to which an "average reasonable person" would commit himself or herself. Subsequently we can allow explicit private contracts to raise or relax those standards. A prospective plaintiff/patient consents (the contract) to relieve defendant providers of their previous obligation (tort law standards).[36] This may appear to violate the central principle I have emphasized, that no assumption of risk can relieve a defendant who has negligently created the risk himself or herself, but it does not. Contractual assumption of risk is really an acknowledgment of an ambiguous area of negligence within which the defense of expense can operate.

Finally we can note how the qualified role of prior consent in setting the basic standard of negligence relieves a lot of the pressure on the difficult question of whether the consent is truly voluntary. The real role for Lamson's, Brown's, or a patient's consent to risk is not subsequent to the determination of a defendant's negligence; their consent's real role is part of the primary issue, the substance of the defendant's negligence. If in the context of determining that negligence it is a plaintiff's presumed consent that is applicable (see conclusion of Chapter 2), whether any choice of the plaintiff was actually free is not a consideration. We only need wonder, as we are imagining this plaintiff's hypothetical, truly free decision, whether he or she would in fact have consented to the risk.

No-Fault Compensation for Accidents of Restraint

But though a defense of expense thus survives proper skepticism about assumption of risk, another huge problem remains. Take our modified fifty-dollar tonometry *Helling* case. Even if the doctor is not negligent, could we not still hold him "strictly liable," as lawyers say?[37] The patient still has to suffer her huge burden of blindness. How can it be fair to leave her uncompensated if she is a victim of sheer bad luck? If we compensated her, however, it would be for a "pure medical accident"—the unlucky result of perfectly proper and justified provider behavior. That would admittedly not seem fair to the doctor. Still, though, if the doctor can spread out the costs of compensation among other patients through malpractice insurance, perhaps having him compensate this patient is right after all.

No matter how we sugarcoat it, such a strict liability conclusion will still be extremely hard to swallow. For one thing, since the doctor was justified in not giving the test, would it not be simply dishonest to have him compensate the plaintiff under the rubric of malpractice? More importantly, how could we reinforce what was in fact his optimal behavior if we hold him liable? As for any injustice in leaving the victims of accidents of medical restraint uncompensated, our convictions here are just not nearly as clear and unanimous as they are about compensating people who have been wronged as well as hurt.

The strongest cases of strict liability, while, of course, by definition they do not involve fault, gain what plausibility they have because defendants have still caused a harm. Causation, however, is largely missing in accidents from justified provider restraint. We could, I suppose, stretch the notion of cause to cover the case in which a nurse or doctor causes an accident by completely justifiably forgoing some item of care. Note, though, that then we would probably have lost the force of our usual conviction that anyone who causes harm is responsible for compensating the victims.[38]

In many cases of strict liability in the law we can call upon subtle traces of background negligence, but these, too, are missing in the case of providers who justifiably forgo excessively expensive care. Blood, for example, is a classic case of possible strict liability where negligence would still actually hide. Courts have usually held that unlike manufacturers under product liability law, hospitals are not liable for the defects of the blood they dispense; either blood is said not to be a product and its transfusion only the dispensing of a service, or it is held exempt from usual product liability because it is "unavoidably unsafe."[39] Both of these lines of reasoning are superficial—product/service is a terribly thin and arbitrary verbal line, and blood is not literally unavoidably unsafe. A much more persuasive argument cuts the other way. Blood presents an ideal instance of economic reasons for liability without fault: blood collection agencies are in a far better position than anyone else to reduce the transmission of disease by obtaining higher-quality blood. Take the problem of serum hepatitis alone. If collection agencies were held strictly liable for its disastrous damage, they would certainly have much greater incentive to procure safer blood.[40]

Thus, strict liability seems efficient if defendants are in the best position to reduce accident costs. Then, however, it is hardly strict—there are traces of potential background negligence. The blood case illustrates that precisely. If we made blood suppliers strictly liable, it would be because we think they can procure a safer supply if they try harder, and given the stakes for real people's lives, it would be efficient for them to try that hard. Precisely because there is some remaining trace of fault we can swallow "almost strict" liability in cases such as blood much more easily than we ever can for strict liability proper. Not only in the name of plaintiff's justice but also in the name of defendant's negligence, blood collection agencies should be liable for serum hepatitis.

All of that interesting analysis for blood, however, does not transfer over into any argument for the strict liability of the doctor in this case. Already, by hypothesis, his behavior is justified and not at all negligent. To generate any conclusion for compensation of the patient we cannot depend on any traces of background negligence. We would have to rely purely on arguments of efficiency or larger distributive justice.

There are some very sophisticated efficiency arguments for strict liability that do merit further examination. By hypothesis, of course, the basic behavior itself, the doctor's restrained use of care, is efficient. The issue is whether it might still be efficient to hold him strictly liable for the accidents that follow. We should probably be more than usually open-minded about this possibility. We usually start thinking about the matter of assigning damages with an unspoken presumption of a fault arrangement: one who suffers harm has to bear its cost unless it is the fault of the injurer. We may then determine the defendant's fault by considerations of efficiency, among other things, allowing a defendant the subsequent response that the plaintiff contributed negligence (a judgment itself, perhaps, determined by efficiency). The upshot of this fault arrangement is that we make the victim bear the costs of accidents not worth anyone's avoiding.

A very different, strict liability arrangement of efficiency and liability is possible, however. We could completely reverse the legal burdens, presuming the injurer to bear the costs of accidents not worth anyone's avoiding. In effect we would be assuming that one who causes harm is liable unless it is really the fault of the plaintiff. In turn, if the plaintiff was at fault, we could allow the plaintiff the defense that the injurer contributed negligence. As long as we defined both parties' negligence by reference to efficiency, these two different arrangements, strict liability and fault, will theoretically be equally efficient.[41]

Any real differences in efficiency between them will then have to rest on other contingencies. A fault arrangement may be more efficient than a strict liability system simply in running fewer cases through the compensation mill.

It will run them through the mill, however, with much higher process costs per case—all those legal battles over the defendant's negligence. And we get back to the other major consideration, previously mentioned, of who is generally in the best position to assess whether the costs of the eventual accidents are greater than the costs of extra prevention.[42]

This is very relevant to the particular context of an extra medical procedure. Who is best positioned to make efficiency assessments, provider or patient? We might at first suspect it is the provider, but that is hardly clear. The nurse, doctor, or hospital administrator is better positioned than the patient to estimate many likelihoods and costs, but the patient can usually say best what those risks mean in his or her own life. On balance it is simply not clear from these minimal and rather obvious observations which general initial presumption of liability—for one who causes harm or for one who suffers it—is more efficient. Strict liability may not be out of the running, but it is hardly in the lead.

An additional factor, however, leans strongly in favor of a fault arrangement except in some prepaid delivery systems. If we hold the doctor liable even for the accidents that result from his proper restraint, we are likely to discourage him from being similarly restrained in the future unless we take some unusual compensating steps. We would somehow have to get him to see that the cost of paying off his victims is still less than the cost of the care he might have otherwise offered. For him to take those cost differences to heart, he needs to feel them, not merely to pass them on to someone else. Only if he is practicing in a prepaid instead of a third-party insurance system is he likely to do this.[43]

In totaling all of this up, we face a maze of different and often conflicting efficiencies. Perhaps nothing definitive can be concluded about the relative efficiency of strict liability as opposed to fault in the gray area of medical accidents where expense might be used as a defense. Most, however, would probably guess that a fault arrangement is more efficient.[44]

That, however, is only efficiency. We are left to consider justice to the plaintiff in deciding whether to compensate the patient. Here the ready comparison is with the explicit social insurance arrangements we have for selected categories of victims—workers' compensation laws, for example. Should the social insurance logic behind such special statutory no-fault arrangements be extended to strict liability in medical tort law?[45] Would strict liability then perhaps make as much sense for accidents from decisions to forgo medical care as it does, say, for workplace accidents?

After careful thought, it is quite clear that it would not make as much sense. There are different, immensely complicating factors in the case of medical restraint. First of all, is tort law the proper vehicle for such commendable compensation functions? To see the point of this doubt, imagine that we have endorsed the social insurance argument for compensating a victim of justified medical restraint. It is essentially no different from the argument for compensating other victims of misfortune (not negligence), so why should tort law not also rescue all other unfortunates? Well, it might be said, let tort law be used to compensate them, too. But it would surely be strange to allow victims of purely impersonal misfortune to gain compensation through tort law. For one thing, whom would they sue? This whole line of discussion simply reveals what may have been suspected all along: a general social insurance fund, not tort law, is the proper vehicle for compensation.

Finally, there is another and even more deciding consideration against strict liability for justified medical restraint. Workers' compensation claims involve difficult judgments about whether an unfortunate outcome happened because of something in the workplace or because of some other factor, but at least we know what it is we are investigating as the possible cause of the accident—the workplace. In the case of strict liability for medical restraint, not even that would be clear. To define the medical restraint that allegedly causes misfortune we need a reasonably clear notion of when alternative medical procedures could have been prescribed. We could say that this happens when any possible procedure that might have helped was passed over by the doctor, but note the incredibly high level of care that strict liability for medical restraint would then enforce. Maybe there is some smaller circle of possible care in relation to which providers in their restraint are strictly liable, but what smaller circle? This is such a difficult problem that it utterly disables any proposal to apply strict liability to the accidents of justified medical restraint. General social insurance programs, not lawsuits, are the much better vehicle for compensating these victims.

All in all, providers have little to fear from strict liability for the inevitable, faultless accidents of correctly restrained care. Strict liability arrangements here would seem to have no final efficiency advantage over fault, and concerns about justice to unfortunate plaintiffs yield little additional support for the case of strict liability. The legal defense of expense remains intact, vitally important for conceptions of medicine's integrity.

NOTES

1. See Chapters 1 and 2 for development of these ideas.
2. These facts are taken from AMA Board of Trustees (1987); AMA Special Task Force (1984); Baily (1985); Gallo (1986); Localio (1985); Reynolds, Rizzo, and Gonzalez (1987);

Seattle Post-Intelligencer, September 1, 1985, pp. F1, F4; and *Seattle Times,* March 10, 1985, p. A3. If the $1.4 million median for infants seems outrageously high, consider a recent $5.6 million award to a nine-year-old Enumclaw, Washington, boy in 1985. Because of mistreatment at birth, Lucas Hollingsworth is brain-damaged and quadriplegic. He cannot walk, talk, or eat by himself and needs round-the-clock attention. With the judgment his parents purchased a house modified to accommodate his handicaps. A therapist is brought into the home four times a week. A trust fund will provide the parents with $2,400 a month as long as they care for him, and Lucas will receive $6,000 a month for twenty years after he is nineteen. See *Seattle Post-Intelligencer,* September 1, 1985, p. F1.

3. For this and figures immediately following, see AMA Special Task Force (1984); Baily (1985); and *Seattle Times,* March 10, 1985, p. A3. All are national figures, 1984.

4. All providers, including hospitals as well as physicians.

5. This is derived from the $10 billion premium figure by the frequently cited statistic that only forty to fifty cents of every premium dollar gets back to patients in the form of compensation. See Danzon (1985a), p. 10.

6. The $10.6 billion figure is from Reynolds, Rizzo, and Gonzalez (1987) and represents 14.1 percent of physician revenues. The $52 billion estimate is from the AMA Special Task Force (1984). In addition the AMA charges that a considerable part of item 1, the premium total, is necessary only because of unjustifiably large awards for pain and suffering, lawyers' contingency fees, awards for punitive damages, frivolous suits, and not subtracting from jury awards what plaintiffs receive from collateral sources of compensation (say, the victim's own insurance) in calculating the damages owed by the defendant. See *Seattle Times,* March 10, 1985, p. A3.

7. This definition is largely from Danzon (1985a), p. 146.

8. One piece of evidence is especially interesting in this respect. A California Medical Association study concluded that 82 percent of iatrogenic injuries stemmed from positive treatment and only 15 percent from incomplete treatment or diagnosis. This makes malpractice suits' stimulation of too many procedures even more costly. See Danzon (1985a), p. 26.

9. All estimates in this paragraph are from Danzon (1985b).

10. The case for a defense of expense is undoubtedly easier to make if we see injury by active treatment as significantly morally different from injury by passive omission. I will try very hard, however, not to resort to any such alleged difference. The action/omission distinction is both morally and legally suspicious, and I want to construct an argument that is better than it.

11. *Eckert* v. *Long Island Railway Company,* 43 N.Y. 502, 3 Am Rep 721 (1871) at 723. One of the tragic details of this case is that since she may have actually been playing on an adjoining track, the child may not have been saved by Eckert's heroism at all.

12. For simplicity I have not mentioned other standard requirements of tort law that are less important to the current discussion—that the defendant's behavior damaged the plaintiff in a measurable way, and so on.

13. I will pursue the strict liability dimension later in this chapter.

14. Judge Learned Hand used what is now known as his famous Hand formula to decide numerous cases. The care demanded of a defendant is the result of "the likelihood that his conduct will injure others, taken with the seriousness of the injury if it happens, and balanced against the interest which he must sacrifice to avoid the risk." *Conway* v. *O'Brien,* 111 F. 2d. 611 (1940) at 612. See also his more frequently cited case, *United States* v. *Carroll Towing,* 159 Fed. Rep. 2d 169 (1947). Hand's opinions may be the most important single inspiration behind the current "economic analysis of law" movement that gives such prominence to economic reasoning. Paradigmatically, see Posner (1977); in particular relation to Hand, pp. 122–24.

15. Washington State Supreme Court, 83 Wa 2d 514, 519 P. 2d 981 (1974). Subsequently, in *Gates* v. *Jensen,* 92 Wn. 2d 246, 595 P. 2d 919 (1979), the Court preserved its earlier

ruling against apparently anti-*Helling* legislation that had been passed by the state legislature in the meantime. It did not overturn the legislation but interpreted it as not really incompatible with *Helling*.

16. For both a concise explanation of this test and its uncritical application to *Helling*, see Schwartz and Komesar (1978).

17. The average jury award for total blindness, 1973 to 1977, as used by Schwartz and Komesar (1978), p. 1283.

18. Intuitively, in fact, that seems roughly correct. Suppose that $1 million is roughly the value of a statistical life generated by people's willingness to pay for safety (see Chapter 3). If people typically think that their lives now blind would be worth somewhere in the range of 50 to 70 percent of the value of their sighted lives, then the value of sight would seem to fall somewhere in the $300,000 to $500,000 range. The matter might be much more complicated than this, however, if we merge into our considerations some of the skeptical questions about QALYs pursued in Chapter 5.

19. Risk aversion: we will pay more than $1 to avoid a 1-in-100 risk of losing $100.

20. Fortess and Kapp (1985), pp. 215–17.

21. Ibid., p. 215.

22. The practical importance of citing a respectable minority view is emphasized by Blumstein (1981), pp. 1397–98. In a different context, whether minimum standards of care for the poor may be lower than the general customary standard, Morreim argues that the respectable minority provision is of no help. Her claim may be correct for that context, but if the basic argument I have tried to construct for this whole book is correct, the general reason she gives should be mistaken: "the law permits only those deviations from custom that maintain or improve patients' health outcomes." See Morreim (1988a), p. 7, and more generally Morreim (1987b), sec. III–C.

23. A suggestive case here, when a few things are read between the lines, is *Wickline* v. *State,* 228 Cal. Rptr. 661 (1986), with later review first granted but then dismissed (231 Cal. Rptr. 560 and 239 Cal. Rptr. 805, 1987). The plaintiff sued California Medicaid (Medi-Cal) for hospital stay regulations and particular judgments in this case that allegedly led to eventual amputation of the plaintiff's leg. The final decision absolving Medi-Cal of liability held that though its regulations and decisions were tight and cost constraining, their results in this particular case were finally supported by the medical judgments of the attending physicians. Medi-Cal did not take away any provider's final prerogative to keep Wickline in the hospital longer. What undoubtedly happened here was that doctors were beginning to shape their medical judgments a bit by the whole context of scarcity reflected in Medi-Cal's regulations.

24. Stern (1983), p. 13. Stern keeps referring to "the constraints of good medical practice" to establish good or bad faith in relation to economic motives without realizing that economic factors can enter at a more fundamental level to determine good medical practice.

25. F. James (1968), p. 192.

26. *Lamson* v. *American Ax and Tool Co.,* 5 NE 585 (Mass. 1900).

27. We may also differ from the court decision in thinking that Lamson's assumption of risk was not truly voluntary or free from duress. See note 31 and accompanying text.

28. *Brown* v. *San Francisco Ball Club,* 222 P. 2d 19 (Ca., 1950), at 20; emphasis added. An important previous baseball case turned in part on whether the defendant was negligent in not screening the section where the plaintiff sat. *Kavafian* v. *Seattle Baseball Club,* 181 Pac Rep 679 (Wash., 1919).

29. Graham (1984), p. 268; and *Rogers* v. *Frush,* 262 A. 2d 549 (Md, 1970), at 554.

30. Atiyah (1982), p. 194.

31. For this sort of analysis of duress, see Fried (1981), pp. 93–102; and Zimmerman (1981). For a slightly different view and many more distinctions about coercion, see Feinberg (1986), pp. 189–262.

32. See Calabresi and Hirschoff (1972), pp. 1065, 1073–74.

33. Bohlen (1906), p. 91; and F. James (1968), pp. 185, 194–96 (my paraphrase). I will assume that this breakdown is roughly correct. I am aware that there are difficulties in parts of it; see, for example, Bayles (1987), 245–49, especially p. 247.

34. See Epstein (1976). In a concrete and moderate vein, see Havighurst (1986). On the more general use of contract in tort law, not just for establishing standards of care, see Atiyah (1986), Epstein (1986), and Robinson (1986).

35. See Danzon (1985a), pp. 209–13, for a sympathetic assessment that emphasizes this weakness and many of the other points in this paragraph.

36. Prosser (1971), p. 440, lists this as one variety of assumption of risk. Here, too, assumption of risk is not a separate defense but an independent component of contract law that touches on tort.

37. Strict liability is liability despite one's lack of fault, liability for an injury simply because it flowed from one's behavior.

38. For a classic, noneconomic defense of strict liability for virtually all harms that one has caused, see Epstein (1980).

39. *Perlmutter* v. *Beth David Hospital,* 123 N.E. 2d 792 (1954); and *McMichael* v. *American Red Cross,* 532 S.W. 2d 7 (Ky., 1975). More broadly, see Burroughs and Edenhofer (1983).

40. Culyer (1977), p. 51. Kessel (1974), p. 270, estimated that the damages from serum hepatitis were $156 per pint of blood, certainly enough to provide collection agencies with an effective incentive to obtain much safer blood.

41. This entire idea is from Calabresi and Hirschoff (1972), pp. 1058–59. Note that *fault* is something of a misnomer for the first arrangement, as if the second held no notions of fault. The second arrangement, strict liability, ultimately allows the attribution of negligence (and therefore fault) to people just as much as the first, but it always does so after an initial presumption of liability without fault.

42. Calabresi and Hirschoff (1972), pp. 1065–69.

43. Of course, no matter what their mode of practice and regardless of whether the legal arrangement is strict liability or fault, malpractice insurance already reduces the degree to which providers feel the costs of accidents. Then note: while malpractice insurance markedly dampens the efficiency incentives of a fault system, it may do precisely the opposite in a strict liability arrangement. With strict liability we worry about losing the power of incentives—if the provider has to pay for the accidents of restraint even when he or she is not negligent, what incentive will he or she have to restrain his care? Liability insurance, however, allows the provider to pass his or her costs through to others, ironically helping the provider to stay efficient.

44. Danzon (1985a), pp. 118–36, 213–27, is less hesitant in declaring fault more efficient.

45. Perhaps the term no-fault should be reserved for explicit social insurance arrangements such as workers' compensation, and strict liability for tort law where a specific injurer is the party who directly pays a claim.

10

Raising Transplants

Scarcity, Not Expense

In 1983, Jamie Fisk and Brandon Hall both grabbed the nation's heart when biliary atresia left them stranded at infancy. Their parents and their pictures pleaded for the right new livers out there somewhere. Also that year a dying mother of four in Michigan found a match, but Medicaid officials refused to pay the more than $150,000 her liver transplant would have cost. They called the procedure experimental, though then and now that label hardly settles the issue. Liver transplant numbers may be small (roughly 200 in 1984, growing rapidly to more than 900 by 1986), but the new immunosuppressant drug cyclosporin has raised the one-year survival rate of this lifesaving procedure to more than 70 percent.[1] That is better than much cancer chemotherapy.

Hearts, too, are part of the transplant picture. In June of 1986, perhaps the most bizarre transplant drama of all unfolded. Two young parents flew from California to New York to plea on Phil Donahue's TV show for a heart for their failing three-week-old baby, Jesse. Midway through the program they heard that the parents of brain-dead Baby Frank in Michigan would give his heart to Jesse—they, too, were an unmarried couple, and they had initially named their baby Jesse. Meanwhile, in Kentucky, Baby Calvin, first in line on the national list when Baby Frank's heart was designated for Jesse, continued his life-or-death wait.[2]

These are only the most dramatic headlines. The far greater dimension of technology's collision with scarcity is the 6,000 to 10,000 kidney patients who currently await transplants. In recent years nearly 9,000 renal transplantations have been performed annually, but many patients just wait—and wait.

169

The shortfall of organs keeps getting worse; the net annual increase in chronic dialysis patients is now 5,000, while kidney transplants grow by only 500. This particular transplant is one of the more effective and costworthy high technologies of medicine, with a roughly 80 percent success rate and distinct quality-of-life and cost advantages over dialysis. But recovery of less than 20 percent of suitable cadaver organs blocks its growth. Tomorrow the same may be true of liver transplants; as their success improves, there could be as many as 40,000 plausible candidates.[3]

While transplanting hearts at $200,000 to $400,000 per patient[4] may not seem particularly cost-effective, especially considering the 80 percent first-year survival rate, they are unquestionably less expensive and produce higher-quality life than the artificial implants that tie patients clumsily to power plants and beds. If it were not for the scarcity of donor hearts, in fact, we might not even be interested in developing the permanent artificial heart. By contrast, if donor hearts were not scarce, the artificial heart's much more modest temporary uses might be truly functional; they could tide a waiting patient over until a suitable donor was found, without thereby ultimately bumping someone else down the line out of a transplant.[5]

Scarcity of organs has allowed us to avoid many of the hard questions about rationing medical resources with which expensive transplant technologies would otherwise confront us. But we should not put the cart before the horse merely because this organ shortage saves us from making hard decisions about the rush of additional expense. Look at the huge real costs of such a strategy—passing over thousands of costworthy kidney transplants, for example.[6]

If we find transplants not worth either their monetary cost or their ethical price in shortcutting consent to obtain sufficient donors, potential recipients cannot complain; not saving them might be unfortunate, but it is hardly unfair.[7] The unfairness charge is plausible, though, if it is so easy for people to donate organs that donation is generally regarded as a duty. Is it fair to let another person die in the prime of life by failing to donate one's organs merely, for example, because one does not like to think about one's death? We need to take a hard look at organ shortage—both at the public policies and at the personal reasons behind the inadequate supply.

In the United States the Uniform Anatomical Gift Act (UAGA) adopted in the 1970s enables people to secure their postmortem donation and authorizes families to donate the deceased's organs when he or she has not consented. This consenting-in arrangement has still left organs in short supply. Few people sign donor cards, and providers hesitate to ask surviving spouses and next-of-kin for permission to remove organs at awkward moments of tragic death. (The most suitable donors are typically young sudden trauma victims.) Recent momentum has developed for a supplementary policy of required request, requiring supervisory personnel at the time of a prospective donor's death to ask next-of-kin for permission.[8]

This supplement may secure something close to an adequate supply, though this is unlikely. If it does not, many will still argue for the UAGA's basic voluntary donation framework. It will be said that to move the next step to an objecting-out procedure—taking organs without people's consent unless they expressly object—would violate patients' and families' liberty, impose on them an inappropriate burden of justifying personal decisions, and show insufficient respect for the body of the deceased.[9]

In this chapter I argue not only that these charges against an objecting-out policy are mistaken but that even if required request can produce for the UAGA a nearly adequate supply of organs, it is misdirected in principle. A variant of the policy of taking cadaver organs unless a donor has objected respects autonomy better than the UAGA's volunteer framework.

In pursuing this issue we must be careful not to use inappropriate labels. Some terms for an objecting-out policy, for example, load the argument against it. *Routine removal* implies that the organs of a person who does not take the initiative to register his or her objection will be automatically extracted; as we will see, however, focusing on objection rather than positive consent leaves open the question of whether the person or the society should carry the burden of registering that state of mind. To speak of *taking* organs unless a person objects is not much better, conjuring up images of a monolithic society grabbing body parts. *Salvaging* and *harvesting* are even worse. Both potentially demean the body—salvaging abandoned or already ruined parts and harvesting a mass of impersonally numerous, undistinguishable items. As catchy as they are, both labels are inaccurate.

Presumed consent is better, but it makes the argument unnecessarily difficult for defenders of objecting out to win. They will feel obligated to show that when people fail to object they really would have consented if they had been asked. But one's failure to object does not necessarily imply one's consent. I will argue something close to the claim that it does, but not precisely: the absence of objection does not so much imply consent as it itself reconciles use of cadaver organs with individual autonomy.

Opting out may avoid all these pejorative connotations, but its counterpart label for the contrasting current American system, *opting in,* loses the moral power of *consent.* In the interest of both accuracy and moral focus I will thus speak of *consenting in* for the current system, *objecting out* for the arrangement I will defend.[10]

Duty, Not Charity

Some of the other language commonly used about transplant organs is also loaded. The paradigm of *donation* is an explicit, conscious gift. That virtually assumes that what we are doing is charity—not our legal or moral duty but a good thing for good people to do.[11] If donating one's organs for transplant is then beyond the call of duty, others should leave it to one to make a private, personal decision about whether to contribute. But what is organ donation, the performance of a moral duty or an act of charitable goodness?

We would probably never want to say that everyone ought to donate his or her organs (those who religiously or conscientiously object, e.g.). That may lead us to think that use of one's organs for transplant is an optional, charitable thing to do, but that simply does not follow. In times of military conscription, for example, we acknowledge that not everyone ought to serve in the military (conscientious objectors, e.g.), yet we do not regard military service as only something people charitably donate. Moral and legal duties can be duties and still have honored exceptions.

The clearest cases of moral duty occur under three conditions: (1) the behavior makes a great difference to someone else—it harms them or blocks some very significant benefit; (2) one's duty must not be so difficult that most people cannot realistically, easily do it—if we have a duty to rescue, for example, it is a duty to relatively easy rescue; (3) some expectation or understanding we have helped to foster creates a special relationship with the person to whom we owe the duty. The clearest examples of things we ought to do that lie beyond the call of duty occur when the last two of these conditions are missing. One person goes very much out of his or her way and drops by for a visit to cheer someone else up, for example, having previously given the second person no expectation whatever that he or she would visit.

Organ donation clearly meets the first two conditions. It confers a huge benefit on someone else, and unless one has religious or ethical objections against it, it is not the least bit difficult to do. For most people it is easy to contribute one's cadaver organs—easy in terms of time, effort, life plans, one's conception of one's other duties, and so on.[12] If, for example, the reason someone fails to donate by signing the back of his or her driver's license is that he or she just doesn't like to think about the possibility of dying, is this not really like the proverbial bystander who lets a blind person walk off a cliff? People who desperately need cadaver organs are admittedly not identifiable at the time of prior donation like the blind pedestrian. But what kind of an excuse is that for not donating organs? It is entirely clear that if the deceased or the survivors fail to contribute the organs, someone will probably die who otherwise would live. If donation is also easy, how can contributing organs be less one's duty than shouting to the blind man?

So two conditions are met. It is usually thought, though, that the third condition of previous understanding or special relationship is missing. This same item is missing in classic examples used to illustrate the difficulty of arguing for a legal duty to rescue. Again, with the proverbial blind man, if one utters not one word of warning as he walks off a cliff ten feet away, is one legally liable? Should one be? Though all can agree at the start that one has a moral duty to warn, the law has traditionally said that there is no legal duty.[13] A legal, not merely moral, duty of easy rescue is tough to articulate in the absense of special relationship.

Right here we are apt to make the important mistake of thinking that since no special relationship obtains in the usual organ donation, defending any policy more restrictive than consenting in must make that very tough argument for a legal duty of easy rescue. That is simply confused. Objecting-out policies impose no legal duties to donate, so we need not defend any legal duty to easy rescue. Objecting-out policies only give an initial legal prerogative to the society, not any right of coercion. People may still object out, with absolutely no burden of justifying their objection. Objecting out thus cannot be described as legal moralism—forcing people to do what they ideally ought to do. It only implies a shift in discussion from "donation" and "charity" to moral "duty."[14]

But while objecting-out policies involve no legal duty to contribute one's organs, we come very close to meeting that difficult third special relationship condition anyhow. Take the organ donation case. At first sight its very nature—contributing for anyone who happens to need organs—seems to preclude any special relationship. Thus, we probably think that using a moral duty of easy rescue to formulate public policy makes general humanitarian altruism into some sort of moral or legal requirement. Duties to rescue, however, can be based on tacit agreements of mutual self-interest, not general altruism. If we are talking about easy rescues of great benefit, it would seem to be in everybody's mutual interest to bind themselves to a universal practice of easy rescue.[15] If people are then also concerned about free riding (beneficiaries of a general practice of easy rescue not performing those rescues themselves), they may even want to make this moral duty of easy rescue into a legal duty as well.

Thus, something much more modest than general altruism is involved in duties of easy rescue. That is certainly true for moral duties and maybe even for legal ones. We confront an implicit contractual relationship between human beings. Admittedly this is not what we normally mean by special relationship—certainly not the one I have with my eighty-year-old aunt, for example, for whom I have grocery shopped the last ten years. But it comes very close to meeting the extra element we are looking for in that third condition of duty. In any case it is sufficient for moral duty.

If prior policymaking contractors consider this in the context of contributing cadaver organs in particular, they will allow anyone with serious objections not to contribute. That is just taking the easy rescue limitation seriously. In practice objecting-out policies can be more generous yet: any objection that people are willing to state can do, without any need to justify it in any way whatsoever.[16]

Ultimately, I suspect, only one consideration can pull reflective contractors back from what is thus actually a lenient objecting-out policy toward some version of consenting in: if we suspect social pressure will cause some people not finally to object, though they want to. Are these pressured acquiescent people a serious enough problem to pull us back to a policy of consenting in? That will depend on the particular conditions of the society; if knuckling under to social pressure is seen more generally to be a significant problem, reflective policymakers might decide that objecting out runs too many risks. But remember that this concern would have to override even the lifesaving advantages of objecting out.

These considerations may make the matter seem complex, but the central point remains simple: we should stop talking—right now, forever—of deciding to allow our transplantable organs to be removed as charitable donation. Though we may be far from legally requiring removal,[17] we need to talk about it in terms of people's moral duty. We should do that even if donating organs does not meet the strong special relationship condition for a legal duty of rescue. Our mutual self-interest in easy rescues meets the weaker version of that condition required for moral duty.[18]

Objecting versus Consenting

Parallel to a moral duty of easy rescue in mutual self-interest, rational self-interested citizens will likely consent to an organ procurement policy of objecting out if it protects the right of unchallenged objection. But this point will not by itself dispense of all criticisms that objecting out is cavalier in handling the dead bodies of free persons. Only voluntaristic consenting in, it will be said, completely respects people's autonomy. Should we not be looking for a person's positive approval, not just the absence of objection?

What is the proper question to potential donors, "Do you consent?" or "Do you object?" These are importantly different queries. Imagine changing the language of patient consent forms generally: "Do you *object* to our taking out half your small intestine?" A query about objection generally seems to presume that the inquiring party is not just neutral. In a therapeutic context the patient is already subordinate in knowledge and power to providers, and it is important not to exacerbate that subordination further. In therapeutic settings there is therefore every reason to ask whether people consent and not whether they object. Is contributing one's cadaver organs while one is still alive any different?

It is. One is not likely to be in the same disadvantageous position vis-à-vis a representative of society who asks one about organ donation as one usually finds oneself in in relation to one's physician. What is the risk in objecting to what some officer behind a driver's-license application desk may seem to suppose by his or her question? Why would the officer take any objection one might choose to express as an affront? We much more naturally expect that a provider might feel affronted by a patient's refusal to accept carefully suggested therapy.

Furthermore, it is crucial to remember here what was concluded in the previous section—that, unless one objects, contributing one's organs is easy and therefore one's moral duty. This provides the most important argument of all for an objecting-out policy. If the stakes of one's decision for transplant recipients are as high as they usually are, failure to consent is not at all the right line to use in carving out exceptions to one's duty. Why should one not have to object, not merely fail to consent, to escape the moral duty to easy rescue? Does one not owe at least that to desperate potential recipients?

Other points are related to this. If the great stakes to others and ease of performance already mean that people have a duty to contribute unless they object, why should we be held back in crafting public policy by any very small increases in the possibility of abuse that an objecting-out policy might involve? A generally effective, good-faith effort to minimize pressure should be morally sufficient.[19]

For objectors it is easy to understand how we might overlook this entire connection of organ procural policy with the usual moral duty to contribute. After all, one then would not have any duty to contribute (one is an objector). Occupying that position, however, can unfortunately lead one to forget that if one did not object, one would indeed have a duty to contribute. A morally sensitive objector will take to heart precisely that fact—the fact that if he or she had no objection, he or she would be morally required to allow his or her organs to be used. But look at what that means: if the objector takes that contingency to heart, will he or she not be willing to carry some small burdens in establishing that he or she does in fact object? Would he or she not admit the responsibility to express any real objections he or she has instead of controlling the situation by mere default?

This also clarifies what an objecting-out policy should do with people who answer that they don't know when they are asked about possible objection. There are plausible things to say on both sides. On the one hand, an "I don't know" response to "Do you object?" indicates a hesitation that leaves providers reluctant to remove organs without further consent. But on the other hand, is that response not sufficient when people are given a clear opportunity to object? If someone really does regard his or her ambivalence as reason enough to block society's use of his or her organs, why should that person not carry the burden of expressing that as an objection? Perhaps in fact the case where "I don't know" really is an objection can be brought out rather easily by a follow-up query: "Does that mean that you would rather not have any of your needed organs removed for transplant?" If after that the person still answers "I don't know," why should providers be seen to have diminished his or her autonomy if they later remove the organs?

We need to be frank about this. To claim that any and all absence of positive consent should control the use of a person's organs says incredibly weak things about our notions of moral responsibility and self-determination. Do rights of self-determination and the moral principle of autonomy warrant the freedom to follow our views no matter how passively we hold or uncourageously we express them? Do the internal workings of self-determination ask absolutely no price from us before moral rights of autonomy kick in? The strength of reaction to these rhetorical questions is most fundamentally why objection and not consent is the proper focus of any public policy on people's organs.

The Burden of Expression

None of this settles the other somewhat different question about who should carry the official burden of stating or recording any objection. Allocating burdens in relation to duties is important in deciding whether consent or objection is the proper state on which to focus, but the burden-of-expression matter goes farther. Who should initiate and record whatever state we decide is the proper focus?

A very strong view of responsibility would not only ask people whether they objected instead of whether they consented; it would also place on them the responsibility to record any objection they might have. At the other end of the spectrum the very weakest view would be to say not only that consent, not objection, is the proper query but that no one should even raise the issue of organ donation with people for fear of pressuring them or invading their privacy. Intermediate arrangements would be for representatives of society to ask as many people as possible whether they object or to ask as many as possible whether they consent.

People usually think of objecting out rather narrowly, as a policy in which it is entirely up to individuals to record their own objection. If that is the kind of objecting-out arrangement we have, then to be on firm moral ground when we use people's cadaver organs after they have not said anything, we would be presuming that if they had been asked they would not have objected. In certain circumstances such a presumption is undoubtedly legitimate, but it is always dubious if actually consulting people was easy (see Chapter 2). And in fact, here it would seem to be so. I suspect we could rather easily devise an inexpensive arrangement for asking most people whether they object to removal of their cadaver organs. We might ask everyone who applies for a driver's license, for example, or whatever other convenient stages could be added to give people the widest opportunity for easy objection. We could also not remove organs when there is any reason for suspecting that people did not have an easy opportunity to object. There is a spectrum of arrangements to choose from here.[20]

The actual reasons people have for failing to contribute their organs color this entire discussion of the legitimate burdens objecting out might place on people who do not want to donate. Several polls have revealed how flaccid are many of the reasons people apparently have for not donating. In Gallup polls of 1983 and 1985 only 25 and 27 percent said they would donate their own kidneys. The reasons are interesting. Fifteen to 18 percent said simply that they "don't like to think about dying," and another significant group said they "never really thought about it." In 1985, 16 percent said they "didn't like the idea of somebody cutting me up." Fifteen percent in 1983 thought "they might do something to me before I am really dead"; in 1985, that response had grown to 23 percent, while 21 percent also said, "I'm afraid the doctors might hasten my death if they needed my organs." Only 7 percent had religious objections, and even though only one-fourth said they would consent themselves, in 1985 more than three-fifths said they would not mind if someone else donated their organs.[21]

Much is probably going on here, but there is no escaping several impressions. Although people have plenty of soft reasons for not explicitly donating, few have firm objections. Looking at this within the conceptual framework of a moral duty of easy rescue, many reasons here seem easy for people to swallow if, though they might object, in fact they choose not to. Furthermore, these responses show that the debate between objecting out and consenting in is no idle discussion. Approaching people to ask whether they object to the removal of their organs is likely to produce quite different responses from asking whether they want to donate. So will making them take the initiative to register their own view compared to being approached by the society.

The significant portion of respondents who feared that providers may not treat patients as faithfully when organs could be removed might also indicate more of a distrust of medical institutions than any final unwillingness to donate.[22] We might decide to acknowledge such relatively passive distrust by placing on the society rather than on the individual more rather than less of the burden to get objections registered. A significant distrust response may also reinforce the original decision that an objecting-out arrangement should not put any kind of reasons test on what constitutes a controlling objection.

No matter how nuanced an objecting-out arrangement might be and no matter how flawlessly it respects the freedom of potential objectors, it will still be seen by some as an extreme means of raising organs for transplant. An unfortunate source of this continuing reaction is a group of otherwise proper hesitations we might call respect for the body. William May, for example, says that having to volunteer forces us to face more clearly than objecting out does the "profound reservations" we have about the use of the body.[23] Leon Kass reminds those he calls the "theorists of personhood, consciousness, and autonomy" of biological debt and the necessity of embodiment. In ceremonious treatment of the dead body we reverently acknowledge this. The body is more than just a tool or incidental precondition of mind. With hands, eyes, tongue, mouth, and lungs, our bodies prepare us for thought. "No wonder, then, that even a corpse still shows the marks of our humanity."[24]

This properly calls attention to the reverence we should have toward the body, but how does it really argue for consenting in? How does having to volunteer force us to face more directly the "profound hesitations" we have about illegitimate uses of the body? Why think that objecting-out arrangements respect the body any less or do violence to it any more than consenting in? Does the immaculately careful removal of a lifesaving organ from the body of a person to whom we have given every opportunity to object count as violence or disrespect? How does an objecting-out policy disrespect one's body if no other aspect of end-of-life ceremonies is changed? Until some answers to these questions are forthcoming, we should say that objecting out can fully respect the body.

As a matter of fact, many countries with long religious traditions of reverence for the body have objecting-out arrangements: Belgium, Denmark, Sweden, Norway, Finland, France, Poland, Hungary, Czechoslovakia, Austria, Italy, Greece, and Israel.[25] Israel's presence on this list is particularly interesting, since orthodox Jews object to autopsy as "mutilation" of the dead.

Even the orthodox Jewish view is that organ transplantation shows no disrespect for the dead and no desecration or mutilation: the contributing person receives no benefit from the dead, there is no delay in burial, and one is contributing to save life.[26]

Thus, we are simply engaging in loose talk about autonomy if we insist that consent is the only proper question contributors should be asked in a free society or that placing a very small burden on people to register their will violates their self-determination. To say that "programs will need to depend on the actual free choices of actual free donors"[27] is no more a defense of consenting in or required request than it is of moderate forms of objecting out. Autonomy and respect allow us to go on and be pulled toward a policy of objecting out by our already admitted duty of easy rescue. The dogged defenders of consenting in have mistakenly stolen the banner of individual liberty and respect right out from under the nose of objecting out. They should not be allowed to get away with it.

Families

How does the dead person's family fit into all of this? I have deferred that question of the proper balance between family and donor prerogatives until now, to be taken up separately.[28]

The question is crucial. The Uniform Anatomical Gift Act currently in force in the United States technically gives a premortem donor control over subsequent objections of the family. Yet even with donors who carry unambiguously signed and witnessed donor cards, the common practice is still to ask the family and not to remove organs unless they consent.[29] It is even more astonishing that this deference to the family in face of clear legal warrant to proceed is found in many countries that have objecting-out arrangements; there, too, providers often end up asking next-of-kin.[30]

The generic term *required request* could be used for any arrangement in which certain parties in the society are legally required to ask about consent,[31] either to the donor when alive or to the family at the time of death. In fact, however, the term has recently come to denote policies requiring hospital officials to ask the family whether they consent to removal of a loved one's organs. Should the family have such a controlling say?

One way of putting this issue is to ask whether one's dead body is in some sense—and in what sense—one's own. The UAGA has explicitly given the predeceased person the right to determine what happens to his or her cadaver organs. The explicit consent that this person records is supposed to override any family objection. The family should simply be courteously informed of the donor's apparent wishes and consulted only about possible evidence that might contradict that apparent consent.[32] This aspect of the UAGA is blatantly violated by the practice of still asking the families of card-carrying donors, but that does not change the fact that the UAGA has already come down clearly on the individual's side of this potential conflict.[33]

In doing this the UAGA has not just said that autonomy is more important than family. Clearly survivors can have very strong wishes on this matter, and they, not the individual, are now alive to experience any frustration of their desires. Just in terms of respecting autonomy, then, why would we give the predeceased person and not the later surviving family control? The UAGA's priority for donor's wishes over those of the family logically requires another claim: the dead body is primarily the property of the deceased. That is why the autonomous desires of the dead person trump even potentially stronger autonomous desires of survivors.

Since property, however, is seldom an all-or-nothing notion (there are always limitations on use), how clear is this sense of the property ownership of our own bodies? The direction of common law rulings on this is rather clear even if certain rulings along the way are hesitant. Does one really own one's body as property? We hesitate; if anything, one seems too close to it to call it properly one's property. To own one's body would seemingly be to call it a thing, but we conceptually associate our bodies intimately with ourselves—persons. And we are not things, or at least we think we should not be treated as things. If we are to suppose that persons are free agents with individual rights and personal dignity, no wonder then that we balk at regarding bodies as property.

The law has occasionally taken this doubt to heart. Courts have sometimes even negotiated control over bodily materials without calling bodies property. In one case, for example, a person's inoperative eyeball was temporarily removed for examination for cancer and mistakenly dropped down an open sink drain in the laboratory. The plaintiff patient won his suit, but the court decided on the basis of his psychological shock upon hearing of the bizarre accident, not on grounds of loss of property.[34]

Although American law has thus hesitated to call live body parts straightforward property, it has consistently called the dead body effectively a person's own property, not the family's.[35] In one case often thought to lean the other way, the deceased had directed that "no funeral services be held for me, and that my body be given to the Dartmouth School of Medicine." When she died the school did not accept her body, and the court ruled that the surviving spouse and next-of-kin had "proprietary rights . . . related to burial." It may look as if this court decided that once a person dies the body is more the property of survivors than of the person, but the court emphasized that "in the ordinary case instructions by the decedent . . . should be respected and followed in preference to opposing wishes of survivors."[36] In other important cases courts have articulated a limited right of the deceased to control what is done with their dead bodies, "as long as that is done within the limits of reason and decency."[37] Certainly organ donation falls within those limits.

Thus, the major thrust of the common law as well as the UAGA is for people's property rights in their own dead bodies. The tradition of family control over the body now speaks only to cases where people have left no specific instructions. Assigning the family the rights to the dead body is largely a way of placing responsibility on them for a decent, respectful burial.[38] The basis of the family's traditional control of the body is respect for the deceased, not the family's right to control the situation if there is a conflict.

All of this runs deeply against the current movement toward requiring request of families. If a person has not left wishes about contributing his or her organs, or if he or she never had any remotely clear wishes about that, family members are undoubtedly the first parties who should be asked. Furthermore, if providers feel so much like vultures in approaching families in tragic, awkward circumstances that we have to make request mandatory if families are going to get regularly consulted, perhaps request should be required. But look at the important opportunity we have already passed up in legislating any of that: consulting the deceased person when he or she was alive. To resort to required request of family without first trying harder to discern the wishes of the decedent is already to imply that the primary prerogatives over the dead body are held by survivors and not the deceased. Not only does this make required request inconsistent with the thrust of the UAGA and common law decisions about control of the dead body, but it shows as well that required request conflicts with considered moral judgment.

Could we supplement an objecting-out policy for the predeceased donor with a later required-request policy for surviving family? This seems less attractive, however, once we break it down into logical alternatives. If the donor has not objected when he or she had the clear opportunity to do so, it hardly seems in order to ask the family in another round. On the other hand, if the person did object, then asking the family is even more out of place. Thus, there is only one circumstance in which resorting to required request of family is defensible, and that is when we have decided that the society, not the predeceased donor, should carry the burden of initiating the inquiry and recording his or her wishes, but when we also suspect that society's representatives have not actually approached the donor.

This shows that if we are going to require request of surviving family, we should at least change the query from one about consent to one about objection. The family could be told, "Since the patient has not recorded any objection, the hospital will follow its official practice of removing vitally needed organs after brain death unless you and the rest of the family object. If you do object, we will respect your wishes." This is actually more humane and less vulturous treatment of distraught survivors than approaching them on the assumption that removing the deceased's organs requires their positive approval.[39]

Required request of family is a step in the right direction; at least it requires something of somebody. The deceased person, though, stands first in line for property rights in the dead body. If he or she has intended surviving family to be the inheritors of that control, then the family's wishes are crucial, but the rights and obligations of survivors are rooted primarily in respect for the deceased, not any basic claims of the family itself. Requiring request of the donor is eminently defensible; requiring request of the family without trying more systematically to discern the donor's wishes is not.

Live Donor Selling

To enlarge supply, we might, of course, try a market. Monetary payment would attract live body and/or cadaver organs from their donors. I will review here some major arguments against live donor selling, briefly extend those arguments to a somewhat different conclusion for a market in cadaver organs, then make some connections back to the choice between consenting in and objecting out.

Over the years an occasional live potential donor has advertised a kidney for sale, or someone desperately needing one has announced his or her willingness to pay.[40] In the early 1980s, such behavior took organized form when Dr. H. Barry Jacobs founded the commercial International Kidney Exchange, Ltd., in Virginia. To save both needy recipients from the disability of chronic dialysis and society from its expense, he proposed recruiting more kidneys with the aid of money: "God gave us two good kidneys. We need only one-half of one . . . to live a normal healthy life. God also gave us the intelligence to perform kidney transplant operations." So why should we not increase our supply of lifesaving kidneys by getting people who would not otherwise volunteer their spare ones to sell them?[41] By the summer of 1984, however, the National Organ Transplant Act banned all sale of body organs. The United States was not alone by any means; France, for example, banned sales in 1976.[42]

There is a real puzzle here. Why should we not be allowed to sell something that we may legally give away for the very same use? Live selling of a second kidney is no more dangerous than live giving—less than a 3 percent risk of serious surgical complications and somewhere around a 1-in-3,000 risk of ultimate fatality.[43] Moreover, though we have legitimate questions about how voluntary some of these sales may be, they are just as voluntary as some of the questionable donations that are permitted. If we overcome our very serious doubts about live related donors' freedom in the emotional pressure of their situation, why can we not overcome our analogous doubts about the freedom of sellers? Then, too, there is an improved result from allowing sales: we can always use more live donors. Although good matches are not essentially easier to achieve with unrelated live than unrelated cadaver donors, live donors often skirt the speed and timing problems that can threaten the success of cadaver transplants. In a situation of marked scarcity, no one is left worse off if voluntary sales are permitted, and some are distinctly better off if supply is thus expanded.

In society's debate we find bad arguments aplenty against the sale of live donor organs.

(1) *Organs only for the rich.* Allowing sale will mean that those who can pay the most will get the best or even the only organs. This simply confuses selling on the supply side of transplant organ use with a full market for both supply and distribution. The typical proposal is only to allow people to sell organs to increase the supply; that sets no precedent at all for allowing them to be distributed on the basis of recipients' willingness to pay. Whatever degree of help society and insurance already now give recipients with the expenses of transplantation could continue if a market for organs on the supply side was permitted.

(2) *Exploitation.* Recruiting organs with money will "plunder . . . poor people's parts for profit."[44] We recoil upon hearing, for example, that poor youth in Queen Elizabeth I's day sold good teeth for fixing into the jaws of the wealthy.[45] In reacting that way, however, are we really objecting to permitting sales or to the desperate general conditions that may motivate poor people to sell their parts? Presumably the latter is true, but then how does society benefit poor people by banning organ sales if it does little about their desperate general conditions?[46]

(3) *Devaluation.* Just as friendship or a person's ethical principles lose value and esteem if they are openly sold, so also will bodily organs. As soon as money enters, valuing something for its own sake goes on the defensive.[47] But bodily organs are not significantly valued for their own sake anyway. Gifts of organs might be valued for their own sake, but that is a different matter. The general citizenry may resonate less to the general organ transplant scene if they understand that a significant number of organs are sold, not given, but how is the value of a lifesaving kidney to its recipient significantly diminished by the fact that it may have been recruited with money?

Moreover, some of these kidneys would not be obtained at all—that is, some of these lives not saved at all—were selling not permitted. Allowing sales should not be proposed to begin with unless it will increase supply.

(4) *Holding out.* When money enters a process of previous nonmarket donation, some sellers will hold out and wring money from desperate recipients or their payors. But though this can easily happen when sellers hold monopolies on their products, how would anything similar occur when we have a multitude of separate live organ sellers? A variant of the argument would claim that deciding not to give so that one can sell and procure a price—any price, even just the "natural" one needed to call forth a given supply—is objectionably holding out on those who might benefit. But that works no better; given the risks that live donation involves, why should one be blamed for asking a price for one's contribution?

(5) *Diminished supply.* Free donations will drop when people are allowed to sell their organs. Donors will come to see giving as forsaking a price they could receive. This argument has been made, for example, against having a supplementary commercial market in blood.[48] The argument is plausible, but if it is factually correct, then defenders of sales as a means to enlarge supply should be the first to abandon their position. Thus, there is no real issue here, only perhaps a factual disagreement. And on the factual score, in fact, the argument seems dubious. In recruiting blood, for example, the United States with a commercial component has not done at all poorly in comparison with the exclusively uncompensated donation systems of most European countries. It is the only industrial nation, for example, to produce an excess of blood for export. Critics can lament the international commercial market in blood all they want, but how does giving-only Britain, for example, stay more saintly when it has to import part of its supply from commercially supplemented systems such as the United States?[49]

These are the bad arguments against live selling. There are other better ones, but they work only if introduction of a commercial market fails to increase supply:

(6) *Virtue.* We feel that a society is a better society and the people in it are more virtuous when their first thoughts run to giving, not to selling. That is an other-things-equal belief, however. If the market did increase supply and more lives were saved by allowing sales, and if people knew that, would we still think that people were really less virtuous in selling?

(7) *Incentives to damage oneself.* Though the final choice to donate a spare kidney and take the risks involved in both the removal procedure itself and doing without a backup should ideally be left to the individual, we still feel uneasy about giving people financial incentive to trade away part of their very bodily security. But since even in selling they are still free agents making deci-

sions about the only real lives they have to live, that worry is minor compared to the value of saving more lives by recruiting organs for a price. If, of course, permitting sales does not enhance supply relative to other ethically acceptable means of procurement, misgivings reappear. Can we in good conscience, for example, ask the living to risk their lives for money because we are afraid to confront our relatively unfounded qualms about objecting out?[50]

The conclusion seems obvious. There is nothing necessarily wrong with selling one's organs if one does it with an open eye, and allowing people to do that might increase the supply of lifesaving organs. But given the moral duty of easy rescue, objecting out is an ethically cleaner option, and it is undoubtedly a more productive one in increasing supply. We are in a moral put-up-or-shut-up situation. We should move to objecting out and thereby save more lives. But if we are not willing to do that, we should at least permit live donor selling to increase supply.

We have been talking about the sale of live donor organs. How does a market in cadaver organs compare? In such a market people while still alive would sell the future rights to their dead body's organs.[51] Again, many of the arguments against such a proposal are bad, including the parallels to the first three cited above. Also, the last argument, the legitimate but limited reservation about giving people incentives to damage themselves, does not apply to cadaver sales.

But one of the poor arguments against live donor sales is much more persuasive when directed against cadavers: the modified version of holding out. Unlike live donations, cadaver donations do not risk the donor's health. Compensation is therefore less necessary to tease them out. But that fact also makes the decision to ask money for cadaver parts instead of donating them stingier than a decision to ask money for contributing spare organs when alive. Barring any serious objection, we have a moral duty to donate cadaver organs, a duty we do not have with genuinely risky live donation. Permitting the sale of cadaver parts would thus allow people to traffick off their blame-worthy stinginess, something we would never say about live donor sales. That would corrupt the benevolent relationship between donors and recipients in a way far beyond what live donor selling ever would.

There is thus a plausible case for banning the sale of cadaver organs. They threaten the larger benevolent relationship between donors and recipients in a way that live sales do not. Furthermore, the ethically acceptable as well as productive alternative of some version of objecting out means that cadaver markets should remain unused.

This is a fortunate conceptual situation. Neither live donor nor cadaver sales are wrong in a way that automatically justifies banning them. Yet, especially in the case of selling cadaver organs, some of the long-run effects are not at all the direction in which most would like to move. We would be headed toward greater self-interest and away from benevolence, solidarity, and gratitude for the lives we have had. Even then, we would be hard pressed to justify banning sales if that meant passing over real lives we could save, but at this point the at least equally productive alternative of objecting out rescues the argument against sales. Like sales, objecting out may appear to constitute a setback for benevolence and gratitude compared to voluntaristic consenting in, but underneath, because it is grounded in the mutual moral duty of easy rescue, objecting out actually reflects greater commitment to solidarity and benevolence.[52]

NOTES

1. A handy summary of numbers and survival rates for major transplant categories is M. James (1988).

2. Chambers (1986). Baby Calvin did get his heart a week later.

3. The figures here are from Caplan (1983), pp. 25, 32; Eggers (1988); Halper (1985), p. 54; Hyman (1981); Iglehart (1983), pp. 125, 128; M. James (1988); Krakauer et al. (1983); Levey, Hou, and Bush (1986), p. 914; Prottas (1985), p. 103; Stuart (1984), pp. 87–89; and Weiland et al. (1984), p. 5. For an assessment of current prospects for lung transplantation, see Baldwin (1988).

4. Per transplanted patient, including the cost of cyclosporin follow-up treatments at $5000 to $7000 per year.

5. On the currently self-defeating effect of the temporary artificial heart, see Annas (1985).

6. The total cost of a kidney transplant in the year in which it is performed is roughly $50,000; 80 percent are successful; ensuing maintenance costs are one-third of those for dialysis, and quality of life is usually better. Eggers (1988).

7. Engelhardt (1984), p. 70.

8. More than half the states have legislated required-request policies, and the federal government has virtually mandated the same thing by requiring hospitals to have proper procedures in place for making inquiries. See 42 U.S. Code 1320 b-8 (1986); and Martyn, Wright, and Clark (1988), pp. 27, 33. For an important early article urging required request, see Caplan (1984).

9. The first sort of objection is reflected in the comment of David Ogden, president of the National Kidney Foundation: taking organs unless people object is "relatively coercive, compared to the more classical freedom of choice that characterizes our way of life." See Ogden (1983). For the second sort of objection, see Gorovitz (1984), p. 9. For the last, see May (1985).

10. The essential objecting-out proposal and even the emphasis on objection is not at all new. One of the early and still most comprehensive and persuasive discussions of this position is Dukeminier (1970). Unfortunately, he used the term *salvaging*.

11. To avoid clumsy, multiword colloquial phrases for good behavior beyond the call of duty, philosophers often use the even clumsier single word *supererogation*. *Virtue* is not clumsy, but it means something different, focusing on the motivation and character of the agent, not the rightness of the action. For important insights on the relationship between supererogation and virtue, see Trianosky (1986). The distinction I am focusing on here is

between duty and charity, not between justice and charity. On the latter distinction, see Buchanan (1987).

12. This is usually true, of course—not when people have decided objections. For more on the natural fit between organ contribution and duty, see Peters (1986b).

13. Vermont and Minnesota have had easy rescue statutes since 1968 and 1971: *Vermont Statutes Annotated,* title 12, sec. 519, supp. 1971; and *Minnesota Statutes Annotated,* v. 38, sec. 604.05 (1985). Two comprehensive prescriptive analyses of the legal duty of easy rescue are Feinberg (1984), pp. 126–86; and Weinrib (1980). Feinberg concentrates on the issue in criminal law statutes, Weinrib more in common law tort; both defend a limited legal duty of clearly easy rescue without resorting to legal moralism (see note 14).

14. Legal moralism means legally requiring something simply because it is morally right—in moderate form, when it is morally required; in extreme form, when it is merely something we ought to do.

15. Lipkin (1983), especially pp. 289–91. This sort of point is used by Muyskens (1978) in arguing for a policy of routine removal of organs.

16. We are led to this simply by the difficulty of devising and implementing any reasons test. It does not indicate that we are backing away from the belief that people have a moral duty to contribute. They do, unless they seriously object. If their objection is not serious, they still have a moral duty to contribute, but because of the difficulty just stated we may decide not to enforce that moral duty in any way in public policy. I am indebted to Ronald Moore for congenial criticism on this point.

17. No U.S. court has required anyone to donate. A noted case on a private request for donation of bone marrow by a living relative is *McFall* v. *Shimp,* 10 D. & C. 3d 90d (1978). In *Head* v. *Colloton,* 331 N.W. 2d 870 (1983), the court denied a plaintiff's request to be told a potential donor's identity so that he could write her a personal appeal.

18. I do not claim that obligations cannot arise in the context of charitable gifts. Murray (1987), pp. 32–34, notes that the relationship between giver and receiver often gives rise to obligations, especially about how to give and receive. But while gift relations involve obligations, the gift act itself is seldom morally obligatory.

19. A similar point has been made by Matas et al. (1985), p. 231.

20. It is interesting to note the varying burdens on providers who remove corneas in states that have some sort of routine-removal/objecting-out statute for corneal tissue in particular. Arizona, Colorado, and Utah require "reasonable search" for the donor's objection and still have to import corneal tissue from other states, whereas Florida, Georgia, Maryland, Michigan, and Texas require only that there be "no known objection" and collect more than they use. See Lambertson (1984). Dougherty (1987), p. 55, notes that the objection condition in an objecting-out policy might be met merely by the decedent's membership in a group known to oppose organ removal.

21. Gallup polls sponsored by the American Council on Transplantation and reported in *Hastings Center Report* (1983), p. 25; and *Tacoma News Tribune,* April 23, 1985, p. A8. See also Childress (1987), p. 89; and for another survey, Manninen and Evans (1985).

22. This is Childress's interpretation (1987), pp. 89–90.

23. May (1985), p. 40.

24. Kass (1985a), pp. 20, 26, 28. Kass, unlike May, does not tip his hand on whether he is therefore opposed to objecting out.

25. Butler (1985), p. 203; Cantaluppi, Scalamogna, and Ponticelli (1984), p. 103; Eliahou (1982); Kennedy (1979), p. 20; Stuart (1981); and *American Medical News,* March 13, 1987, p. 46.

26. Schwartz (1984), p. 423. I am tempted to say that Israel's example should put to rest once and for all any criticism that objecting out does not show proper respect for the body. I wonder how May would explain his hesitations to an orthodox rabbi.

27. Engelhardt (1986), p. 366.

28. In devising final real policy, of course, consent versus objection and society versus individual burden-of-expression choices have to be made together with the family-versus-donor choice. Some of the combinations get very complicated. Take, for example, Great Britain's legal arrangement. Consenting in governs what the society may do in relation to the donor's own wishes. If the donor has signed a donor card, those wishes trump any objections the family may have. If the donor has not signed, providers in control of the body at the time of death may remove useful organs, provided they have made a "reasonable effort" to contact next-of-kin about their consent and have failed. If next-of-kin either take their own initiative to object or do not consent when contacted, organs may not be removed. See Pallis (1982), p. 336; and Miller (1985).

29. Prottas (1985), p. 101.

30. Cantaluppi, Scalamogna, and Ponticelli (1984), p. 102. This and the low sensitivity of providers to the need to pick out potential donors explain why countries with objecting-out arrangements currently also fail to meet their needs for cadaver organs.

31. Or even, theoretically, about objection, though then the required request label would be odd.

32. States already doing this are California, Colorado, Florida, and Wyoming. Overcast et al. (1984), p. 1560.

33. Peters (1986a), p. 242. Peters also points out a gaping inconsistency in the UAGA: people who object to removal have no way of preventing their families from donating their organs. If the conflict between one's stated wish to donate and one's family's objection is settled in one's favor, why should not a conflict between one's expressed objection and the family's wish to donate also be settled in one's favor?

34. *Mokry* v. *University of Texas Health Science Center at Dallas,* 529 S.W. 2d 802 (1975). With some of the same conceptual skepticism about the body and body parts being property, most courts have ruled that product liability law does not attach to blood. The selling and dispensing of blood is only a service, rather than blood itself being property, a product of the body, or a commodity. Hospitals, blood banks, and donors have thus not been liable for the damages of defective blood on the same strict basis as product liability. See Scott (1981), pp. 192–93; and Dickens (1977), pp. 195–96. A leading case for the view that blood is not a product is *Perlmutter* v. *Beth David Hospital,* 123 NE 2d 792 (New York, 1954). Ireland (1973) mounts a persuasive argument against this whole service-not-product position. Generally, see also Lipton (1986).

35. The historical background of the status of the dead body in Anglo-American law is interesting. In the early 1600s, Lord Coke crystallized the law for the next several centuries. Since *cadaver* means "flesh given to worms," he said, no one had any property rights in a corpse. In 1856, the New York State Supreme Court called Coke's linguistic bluff—how could etymology dictate legal substance by itself? It ruled that disturbance of a dead man's graveyard violated something very like his daughter's property rights in his corpse. See Note (1974), p. 1241.

36. *Holland* v. *Metalious,* 198 A. 2d 654 (1964).

37. *Matter of the Estate of Moyer,* 577 P. 2d 108 (1978).

38. Peters (1986a).

39. I owe this observation and most of the way I have put this revised approach to the family to Muyskens (1987). Some of the reservations about required request by Martyn, Wright, and Clark (1988) would also be handled by change from a request for consent to an inquiry about objection. In response to Martyn, Wright, and Clark, see Caplan (1988).

40. For advertisement by a donor, see the December 25, 1983, *Burlington County Times* (N.J.), quoted by Annas (1984), p. 23. For advertisement by a buyer, see Brams (1977), p. 187.

41. Explanatory material distributed by Jacobs' International Kidney Exchange, Reston, Virginia, 1984.

42. U.S. National Organ Transplant Act, title 42, para. 274e; Pub. L. 98–507, title III, para. 301, October 19, 1984. For the French legislation of December 22, 1976, Article III, see Farfor (1977), p. 4; and Broyer (1982), p. 342.

43. The point here is from Andrews (1986), p. 32. The risk figures are from Blohme, Gabel, and Brynger (1981); Levey, Hou, and Bush (1986), p. 915; and Weiland et al. (1984), p. 6.

44. Gorovitz (1984), p. 11.

45. Dickens (1977), p. 159.

46. Andrews (1986), p. 32.

47. This general point outside the context of organ procurement is powerfully articulated by Kelman (1984), pp. 61–72.

48. This was part of the larger case that Titmuss (1971) built against commercial markets in blood.

49. Sapolsky (1984), p. 815; see also Drake, Finkelstein, and Sapolsky (1982). For the contrary attack against the international market in blood, see Hagen (1982).

50. A similar point without reference to objecting out is made by Starzl (1985).

51. I suspect there are particularly strong convictions that other people—family members, for example—should not make money off the deceased person's body without that person's consent. For the many variations of how to arrange a market in cadaver organs, see Peters (1984). A detailed articulation of one proposal is Schwindt and Vining (1986). For a general defense, see Manga (1987).

52. In developing my thoughts on this entire issue I am especially indebted to David A. Peters. I have not taken up one option that Peters (1988) has begun to write about in detail and that Childress (1987) and Muyskens (1987) have also treated: linking organ procurement and distribution, so that only those who have consented to donate their own cadaver organs are eligible for receipt. See Borna and Mantripragada (1987) for a similar "barter" system. Such arrangements could be fair but I suspect would not be preferable to objecting out. They do not highlight the important general moral duty of easy rescue that underlies objecting out, and in the form in which Peters argues for them they require us to make the difficult distinction between valid religious reasons for not consenting and weaker ones. Furthermore, there are problems in maintaining a legal duty to contribute, so we have to fall back on just a moral duty to contribute. But how can we make such a crucial thing as eligibility for receipt contingent on carrying out one's moral duty to contribute, without making the whole arrangement more moralistic than a system with clear and easy opportunity to object out would ever be?

11

The Duty to Die Cheaply

Disturbing Costs

Americans spend roughly 10 percent of their health-care dollars and more than 1 percent of their GNP on health care for elderly people in their last year of life.[1] Other estimates seem even higher: for all ages, 18 percent of medical expenses are run up in the last year of life, 12 percent in the last month. More than 20 percent of health-care monies are spent on patients who are in some sense "terminally" ill.[2] Nearly 30 percent of Medicare's dollars are spent by the 6 percent of its enrollees who die in a given year, and in turn 5 percent of those cost Medicare more than $30,000 each. Already in 1983, the average American dying of cancer incurred $22,000 of expenses in his or her final year of life. In addition to these averages, of course, one finds individual cases and disease categories for which the expenses of dying run much higher. A $100,000 bill would be the norm for several months in a hospital. In-center dialysis for kidney failure is $35,000 per year. Total care for AIDS victims averages $150,000, for only fifteen months of life remaining after diagnosis.[3]

Some fundamental disease and population trends add to the alarm about the future of medical costs. Health-care expenditures are shifting from acute to chronic diseases and from younger to older patients. Some observers have called this the age of delayed degenerative diseases. We have managed to postpone the onset of many chronic diseases, but because we have also extended longevity we have not realized our hopes for "squaring the curve"—reducing chronic diseases so that people live with less illness and die more "natural deaths."[4] We have not really reduced disease, just shifted its character and timing. It begins to seem that no matter how much we progress medically, we may never halt the increase of health-care bills in old age.

All of this is reflected in increasing talk of the high cost of dying and infamous suggestions such as those attributed to former Colorado governor Richard Lamm that the terminally ill have a "duty to die" and get "out of the way." I will strongly defend one restricted sense of such a duty, but it is important not to be carried away with wild misconceptions of the problem's economic dimensions.

For example, although 5 percent of those who die with Medicare coverage incur more than $30,000 of expenses during their last year of life, the percentage of total Medicare recipients who die in a given year is small enough that entirely eliminating those $30,000-plus cases would only save 4 percent of the Medicare budget.[5] More importantly, these figures about the high cost of dying may be more frightening than relevant. For one thing, unless we have some knowledge beforehand about who among those who might be treated is going to die anyhow, how can we avoid these high costs? Furthermore, as the Medicare figure just noted indicates, attacking the high costs of dying for the few who run them up will not by itself make a huge dent in health-care costs.

As salient as they are, however, these corrective points do not erase the real concerns about the use of valuable resources. For a wide range of cases we loosely label terminal, decisions to use or forgo expensive care still represent important occasions for conservation of valuable resources. One of the more common sorts of situation involves hospital intensive care. The British, for example, use it at less than a fifth the frequency of Americans. If Americans could use it even marginally less frequently, medical costs could be reduced by billions of dollars.[6] With regard to hospice care, conventional hospital care is more than twice as expensive, so when hospice is an equally palliative (though perhaps slightly less life-prolonging) option, should the patient even be offered hospital care as an option?[7]

Suggestions here that we have a duty to die to conserve resources or that our end-of-life care should even be rationed raise tremendous resistance from traditional identification with the sick, old, and dying. Unless we have rationed health care in every other area first, how can we even think of picking on these most vulnerable of citizens? The terminally ill are already in the most unfortunate of all human conditions—dying. Would rationing at the end of life not smack of an economic investment motif that will inevitably stigmatize the dying and elderly as second-class, nonproductive citizens?[8]

In this chapter I argue against that traditional resistance. For one thing, the economic investment warning, as relevant as it is in many contexts, is here simply misplaced. Productivity is not the issue at all; as a possibility to be considered seriously, rationing does not emerge from the fact that elderly patients are not productive economically but simply from doubts about whether the extent of the actual benefit of life achieved by their care is worth its expense. No nonproducer stigma has to be operating here at all.

More specifically, I argue that people have a personal moral duty to conserve resources in the courses of treatment they choose for their dying. Then I will pick up increasingly complicated and controversial possibilities: rationing terminal care (in effect, imposing the performance of such a duty) and rationing quasi-terminal or low-benefit nonterminal care in old age.

A Personal Moral Duty

Opinions that the dying ought to die more quickly than slowly are anything but new. Plato, for instance, held that people who were chronically ill and could not return to work ought to refuse medical treatment.[9] Nietzsche wrote that doctors should give, not prescriptions, but a "fresh dose of disgust" to sick people who "continue to vegetate in a state of cowardly dependence."[10]

Recent history has been dominated by a very different idea: the so-called right-to-die. Historically this right was a virtually inevitable reaction to a medical profession that was less than attentive to patients as persons and insurance arrangements that made cost no object. Medicine just did what it was wont to do, including keeping people alive even when living longer was no real human benefit. Against all this it was inevitable that sooner or later we would assert a right to die, a right that would come into play when it seemed that the benefits of treatment were not worth the pain, suffering, or dependence involved. Note that the question of whether, when there is some net benefit for the patient, there is enough to justify the expense does not come into play in this right-to-die framework.

The right to die is now legally well entrenched. Competent patients generally have a right of informed consent, perhaps more transparently stated as a right of informed refusal. In the 1970s, this right got more and more clearly applied to terminally ill patients. In the mid-1970s, the right to die also got extended to incompetent patients who had no chance of recovery. Being incompetent was no longer any reason to deny a person the opportunity to exercise his or her right to refuse treatment. Society just has to decide what other people are best situated to interpolate what that incompetent patient would have wanted, then allow them to decide.[11] Of assistance to patients in thus controlling their dying destinies are legal devices such as advance directives (living wills) and durable power of attorney.

A major reservation in the entire business of conceiving and implementing the right to die has been the fear that it might subtly, socially coerce people into dying before they really wanted to. Some "right to life" groups have extended this worry into wholesale opposition to living-will legislation. Many others, more moderate, have at least thought that precisely what we must guard against in promoting the right to die is sliding toward thinking that people have any duty to die. After all, society could use such a duty to exert powerful social control on dying patients' decisions. Then the dying would be living only by the permission of others, not by their own rights. Images of society or vulturous relatives manipulating away a patient's very life so that society could retain farm price supports and MX missiles or so that relatives could have second chickens in their pots keep this caution very much alive.

Reservations here have probably not slowed down the growing acceptance of the right to die itself, but they have set clear conceptual limits for what we think is proper in decisions about allowing people to die. About a dying uncle, for example, we are apt to feel ashamed if we catch ourselves as relatives, taxpayers, or fellow insurance subscribers thinking or saying that we do not want to help pay any more for extending his life. Above all, we think we should not foist off on the uncle himself the burden of thinking about the financial dimensions of prolonging his dying.

But ultimately such limits on thinking simply constitute not owning up to hard decisions about scarce resources. Imagine what an honest uncle himself might say could he get in on our thoughts. "Stop pampering me and let me say something. I understand your concern about cost—I wouldn't want to pay for your death-prolonging care were you in my current fix, so why should you feel bad about not wanting to pay for mine? In fact," he might continue, "I wish we'd all talked about this ahead of time, like even before my parents and aunts and uncles were dying in their hospital beds." All of us would be better off in the long run if we would have agreed that sometimes even when there is still net value left in life, we should let people die. We should ask ourselves whether it is not our own unwillingness to confront the issue, not our uncle's, that leaves us still hanging with the limp conviction that we should never think people have a duty to die because of expense.

Thus, it seems entirely clear that some sort of duty to die cheaply is thinkable. Should we finally endorse it, however, and actually think in terms of such a duty? Maybe dying more quickly than slowly because of expense is good and admirable behavior, but on the scale of moral urgency does it not fall far short of duty—heroic, say, but not morally required?

The usual conception of a moral duty to contribute to the welfare of others generally requires that one's cost in performing the duty be minor and its benefits for others great.[12] Admittedly, the second condition is met here: the benefit that could accrue to others if resources now used for one's dying were to become available for their more vital uses is often great. Still, if life is the benefit one would be giving up, the cost to one is hardly minor. How, then, can one see forgoing a part of one's life to save expense as a duty rather than action above and beyond its call?

That, however, hardly destroys the case for holding on to duty. For one thing, in many realistic cases the additional life in question is hardly major. If the quality of life, for example, is already compromised to the point where real, considered attachment to it has diminished, we would be blind and simplistic to continue to lump any and all preservation of life into the great benefit bag. Even when it is still a benefit, it can be a very slim one. The segment of life in question also often comes at a stage where one ought to be more ready for death than before.

Furthermore, sacrificing the benefit of time in life might be attended by a compensating positive benefit of knowing that one is parting with a small share of life for the benefit of others. In this respect Daniel Callahan in *Setting Limits* has raised a point of great potential significance: people can create much more meaningful last stages of their lives if they see themselves passing on the torch of life to subsequent generations.[13] The point is not that the added meaning derived from contributing to others by itself creates the duty to die cheaply. For that duty to exist, independently and already the portion of life forgone must not be of great importance to the individual; otherwise we would be saying that those individuals who admirably find their lives more meaningful from contributing something significant to others are morally duty-bound to part with life, while others with less admirable characters have no such duty. How could that be fair? What this newfound meaning for our lives can do, though, is cushion second thoughts we may have—doubts that our sacrifice of additional life is too high a final price to pay for helping others.

Such a duty to die cheaply is strengthened by another, quasi-contractual element. If preserving lives of declining quality in old age is much less a benefit to the aged patient than the resources saved can be for others, then it will be in the mutual self-interest of all to have a general practice of letting death come more efficiently. But if we can actually stick to such a practice, then it is downright selfish now, when one is dying, to cling to every last bit of one's life at great expense. We ought to call such behavior by its right name: a selfish violation of the duty of mutual aid, the duty not to use up more than one's share of the pool of common resources.

The "one's share" condition, of course, is crucial, for one is perfectly well permitted to use resources up to that share without in any way violating one's moral duties to others. But the borderlines of what is one's share are already a function of the minimal benefits of the marginal care in question and one's consequent willingness to adopt a social practice of regarding the sacrifice of those benefits as a requirement of duty and not a merely optional, virtuous act. If one has led a reasonably full life already and there are considerably more beneficial uses to which such resources can be put, is one really, honestly prepared to argue that those resources are still one's share?

A common misconception here is for dying people to think that the resources are simply, straightforwardly theirs. At the start of this whole discussion we can say only that they belong to the Medicare fund or the insurance pool. To parts of these funds, of course, dying patients do have certain rights, moral and/or legal. But just what those parts and rights are is precisely what we are arguing over here. It would clearly beg the basic question at issue in dying patients' favor to insist at the start on their right to use the pool's resources to extend their lives when that benefited them much less than alternative uses could help others.

If all this is correct, I see no other conclusion than to bite the moral bullet and commonsensically say that allowing oneself to die to save resources can indeed be one's moral duty. Mary Rose Barrington envisioned a culture with just this sort of perception: "What if a time came when . . . the decision to live on for the maximum number of years were considered a mark of heedless egoism?"[14] We might wish to withdraw "heedless" from her statement of the point, but she seems to be otherwise right on the mark. We have often admired people who hang on to life as heroic, or reflecting the sacredness of life, but in our increasingly acknowledged context of scarce and pooled resources, isn't *egoism* the typically more accurate label? Why should we not talk as much of being selfish or crass about life itself as about all the other things that people can be selfish or crass about? If after a reasonably long and complete life one refuses to "get out of the way," that may not be admirable individual determination but moral weakness, allowing technologies to detour one from the course to which one previously found it in one's interest to consent.

So let's just take a few of the gloves off our moral language here: dying more cheaply and less expensively is not just admirable sacrifice; sometimes it is morally required. Just as we serve our own vanity and distort moral reality if we speak of the person who only stops by the roadside or gives to Oxfam as a saint or hero, so also we corrupt ourselves if we think that refusing to allow sizable resources to be spent chasing after a bit more of life is heroism. We may just be doing our duty.

A vigorous reinforcement of this point can come from theological perspectives. As Eys and Vaux put it, "our obsession with personal health alienates us from the world and denies God's sovereignty over us." When we reject even relatively wholesome aging as losing health, we have defined health as complete personal freedom from abnormality and lost sight of the larger biological scene, making idols out of ourselves.[15] It is simply bad stewardship to forget about how these resources could be used for other things on earth just because, with insurance, little of the immediate cost hits us in the pocket.

One might think that speaking so bluntly of duties rather than only of rights to die brings us dangerously close to taking choice out of the hands of the dying person and giving it to someone else—state, hospital, insurance plan, doctor, relatives. But by itself, speaking of duty simply does not do that. We call many of our actions moral duty without legally requiring and enforcing them. If, having solidified our convictions about people's right to be allowed to die, we go on to the fleshier language of moral duty, we have not proposed any legal, state-enforced duty at all.

Even in its relatively weak form—personal moral duty—this duty is not impotent. There are many situations in which dying people are still competent to exercise some decisive control over these choices, and, above all, there are plenty of things one can do to facilitate stewardly action should one become incompetent. When we conceive of many of these decisions as duty instead of mere virtue, we will have to attend much more carefully to the future of these matters for ourselves. How many families keep prolonging their loved one's life largely because they cannot bear their own self-perceived guilt in letting that person die? Each and every one of us should see ourselves as having the responsibility to nip these problems in the bud. We ourselves can best dissolve the potential guilt that might immobilize our children and spouses if we fall incompetent. If our relatives are queasy about these matters, we must express our convictions to them now before we can no longer do so.

Rationing Terminal Care

I have stressed that having such a personal moral duty to die cheaply is hardly yet rationing—that would be living under an enforced duty. Yet it would be naive to act as if none of the considerations that press toward personal moral duty constituted pressures toward removing people's immediate freedom of choice. Of course there is momentum in that direction. It is highly likely that in situations of terminal illness, life-prolonging as distinct from palliative care falls far down the scale of real human benefit and thus low in any sequence of cost-benefit ratios. If we are doing any significant rationing at all in order to achieve greater overall efficiency, some terminal care is very likely going to be a prime candidate for cuts.[16]

The reason for this, too, is not just mindless social forces. To have resources for more valuable uses, we would be willing to bind ourselves beforehand to limitations on the least beneficial items in the system. If such prior consent, presumed or actual, works to justify rationing of any beneficial care, it would certainly seem to work in the case of relatively low-benefit, high-cost, life-prolonging terminal care.

What we clearly will not commit ourselves to doing without is palliative terminal care. If anyone traded away his or her right to that kind of care, the rest of us might even refuse to follow through on the bargain; maybe "it would be socially offensive to have to watch the terminally ill . . . suffer from lack of analgesics or lie in filth."[17] Basically, though, that is beside the point. We need not even reach such an objection. Unless palliative terminal care is incredibly expensive or the need for it very short-term, virtually no foresightful subscriber would cut it short in any prior allocation arrangement. People who worry that rationing care for the terminally ill will commit us to denying them palliative measures forget the prior consent rationale for rationing.[18]

There are, to be sure, other objections to seeing people's consent as justifying rationing care at the end of life, but they, too, are not persuasive. Precommitment is sometimes read as a kind of ambivalence, for example. If we really were sure of our choices, Daniel Wikler writes, why would we need to bind our later choices? Is not the fact that we suspect we might later change our minds itself an acknowledgment that our will just does not have a clear direction?[19]

It could be. But as a general point, this argument, too, is a misunderstanding. It misses the peculiar problem contributed by insurance to the whole scenario in which we plausibly come to think of rationing as necessary. If our last-minute wish to employ life-prolonging care at death's doorstep indicated a genuine opinion that overall its benefits warranted its costs, then, yes, the strain with any earlier precommitment would indicate true ambivalence. But insurance makes it probable that we will often voice those later wishes from a fundamentally different orientation: once significantly insured, we think we can ignore care's cost-benefit ratio. That may be especially true at the end of life when we will not live long enough even to suffer the tiny rise in premiums caused by our particular use of the care in question.

To be sure, precommitment can be abused by people who do not seriously reflect on their terminal futures, but how can ignoring the distortion of cost-benefit judgment clearly occasioned by insurance constitute any kind of satisfactory response? We might indeed discard the choice of a thirty-year-old not to invest in any policy that provides care prolonging life from eighty-five years of age to eighty-five and a half. Living that extra half-year at eighty-five probably seems very unimportant to one at thirty, and that is reason enough to take a thirty-year-old's perspective on old-age policy with a grain of salt.[20] But none of that is reason to take the eighty-five-year-old's word as controlling, either. The terminally ill elderly person is apt to forget the relatively low time-in-life benefit of life-prolonging care at that stage. We keep coming back to the critical role that those relatively low benefit payoffs play in any more comprehensively envisioned, nontemporally confined reasoning.[21]

This sort of prior consent defense of rationing life-prolonging care does not have to involve another moral argument often made for age differences: the eighty-five-year-old, it will be said, has a weaker claim simply because, being eighty-five, she has already had a shot at the good things of life. Let's call this the lifetime equality argument for age-rationing. Regardless of whether life extension in old age comes up short on any such yardstick of justice and opportunity, the earlier point still holds: the relatively low benefits achieved by expensive death-delaying terminal care make it an early candidate for rationing. Thus, any limitations of that justice-and-opportunity point are less than damaging to the case for rationing terminal care.

Robert Veatch, for example, argues that "lifetime equality" loses much of its force in terminal illness situations: "Some needs of persons are so immediate that they command attention regardless of the amount of wellbeing experienced over a lifetime. . . . For some care the immediateness of the need is morally overpowering. . . . Equality at that moment in time is what is required."[22] But for what terminal care is the immediateness of need morally overpowering? Palliative and basic nursing care, of course—in general, in fact, the care that we have already not downgraded in importance in any of our prior consent reasoning. But if it is proposed that high cost-benefit, life-prolonging measures also go on that list of more protected care, we have our doubts. From any more time-neutral perspective we identify much less with terminal life extension than we do with minimizing morbidity and suffering.

Suppose we accept the general idea of rationing expensive terminal care that provides only a shot at short reprieves from death. What actual form could such rationing take? If we are unimaginative about its prospect, we might think only of rather unpalatable scenarios such as rigid cutoffs of any and all life-extending care once patients are pronounced terminal—or, worse, rigid cutoffs at age sixty-five. Clearly there are more acceptable methods of rationing. For one thing, adjustments can be made for the importance to particular patients of that remaining small addition to life. Why should factors with which we can widely identify, such as the imminent return of a close friend or relative from a far-off part of the world or the quick approach of Christmas with its family reunion, not make a real difference? There are a variety of such relevant personal circumstances that very much affect the real benefit of the extra life that might be bought. What should not be allowed to sway us, however, are blind, across-the-board convictions that life must always be pursued at all cost. People may have every right to choose expensive private plans ahead of time and pay more for such a care-in-any-circumstance approach, but we are quickly reaching a point at which such views are not common enough properly to control public programs such as Medicare.

If we get along without rigid formulas to determine when people get only palliative terminal care, however, we need not leave all decisions to individual practitioners and circumstances. Institutional decisions can nudge behavior in a more conservative direction: just not having as many ICU or hospital beds, and building more palliative care facilities if in fact they offer their alleged financial saving. If it is the general sense of a hospital's personnel and clientele, for example, that a noticeable number of ICU or general ward bed days are going for marginal care, then the institution should not sit on its hands. It should assist its personnel with concrete encouragement for more conservative decisions by tightening up on supply, a situation that practitioners will quickly learn to take into account. A cooperative approach is possible. Neither hospitals nor physicians should be passing the buck to each other.

Quasi-Terminal Care

True age-rationing, of course, would not confine its limitations to lower-benefit categories of care. When one reached the appropriate age, that itself would determine that life-extending care would now become lower priority. It is not surprising that we resist such proposals, for they seem to imply that even when segments of life bought after a certain age are rather long and personally well appreciated, they are less valuable. Even from the earlier perspective of persons trying to make tough saving and allocation decisions for the resources of our whole lives, it is doubtful we will just throw all life-extending care after a given age into the same low-priority bag. "If I get there," we think, "maybe it will be my most appreciated time in my life." If we are going to ration care at all in old age, almost all of us would probably prefer to ration by the relevant characteristics of care in old age, not by age itself.

An appearance of rationing by age per se is probably what strikes many people as objectionable about British kidney dialysis policy. No one over age sixty-five, we hear, gets that treatment. Thirty percent of European dialysis centers indeed exclude patients older than sixty-five.[23] The question, though, is whether that practice is really intended to exclude prospectively stable, long-term dialysis patients. If it is, and if dialysis for those patients is not just seen to be more expensive per benefit achieved than care already forgone in other parts of the system, then British practice would be an example of real age-rationing.

But is it? We might see dialysis for such patients as virtually always occupying a lower ranking because of its quasi-terminal character (it might work, but only, say, for a few years), or the real drop in the value of the life it adds, given the complications that frequently occur. If either of these factors is present in the bulk of actual situations, denial of dialysis is hardly just a stigmatizing affront to patients as "old" and "dispensable." With these two factors in mind, would people not be likely to consent beforehand to policies of denial?[24]

We might, of course, think that the perception that the life dialysis adds is diminished in quality is itself biased against patients on dialysis. There is, though, some objective basis for this perception. A significant number of patients themselves reject dialysis.[25] Apparently they believe that the added life dialysis could bring is either so short or so low in quality that its net value to them is essentially zero. If that is what is really going on in their rejection of dialysis, and if those who thus reject the treatment are already significant in number, undoubtedly many kidney-failure patients get low enough value from the added life of dialysis that though they do not reject it, it clearly becomes a first-order candidate for rationing. After all, in-center dialysis, at least, is a $30,000-per-year therapy.

We should also be frank about the value of certain other sorts of life with which old age may confront us though the situations may not be terminal. Extending severely demented and senescent patients' lives should have lower priority even if their lives have no predictable limit. Some may even see the relatively common development of senility near the end of life as a sort of terminal illness underneath, even if people don't literally die from it; after all, it's a clear sign of an approaching end.[26] That view is misleading, for the far more important and immediate consideration is simply that the life is severely demented. That may not be morally significant if we are dealing with patients who have never been competent their whole lives. But when the dementia falls at the end of a long and richer sort of existence, most people trying to think out how to use a limited set of resources for themselves do lower the relative importance of such a period of life. I think it is virtually unquestionable that the real individuals of our society, if they really had to make such a judgment for themselves, would regard life-extending care for the severely demented as very low in priority indeed.[27] Is it not literally crazy to forgo life-extending care for other kinds and stages of life before cutting out life-prolonging care for the severely demented? Like low-benefit terminal care, life-extending care of the severely demented becomes a first-order candidate for restrictions if we take seriously the task of matching rationing policies with people's actual values.

In all of this, the situation of facing rationing trade-offs is what finally convinces us that it is sensible to limit some of these nonterminal categories of care. Thinking in that framework, we may well decide to ration nonterminal dialysis, for example, if we see it stacking up as comparatively low-benefit care. By contrast, we will almost certainly give chronic, long-term care for the elderly distinctly higher priority in any such trade-off context. If we think at all clearly, we will not end up abandoning the elderly to waste away in misery.[28]

The only way out of this argument is to deny that we should think about providing health care as a matter of hard trade-offs among relative priorities. But in effect, we already decided to engage in that difficult game when we adopted a public program such as Medicare for the bulk of medical care for the aged. Since then the context of considerations about medical care for the elderly has necessarily become what we might call congressional—seeing ourselves as responsible legislators. Unless we are prepared to retract that basic decision that old-age care should be largely publicly funded, it is plainly irresponsible to ignore trade-offs among all the various functions to which public monies might be put. Suppose we are faced with drastically underfunded prenatal care programs, for example, that are also within the province of government support. It would then be utterly irresponsible of us to refuse to put less important resource uses on the trading block. Do we really care enough about open-heart surgery for ourselves at age seventy-five to continue paying for it but refuse funding for better prenatal care? To duck this problem when we have already decided to finance health care for the elderly and indigent with public funds would simply be burying our heads in the sand.

A society with integrity will not run from these responsibilities. Strong providers and patients will not run from them either.

NOTES

1. Fuchs (1984a), pp. 163–64.

2. Fries (1988), p. 423; and Scitovsky and Capron (1986), respectively.

3. Except for those cited in notes 1 and 2, the figures in this paragraph are drawn from Kovar (1986), p. 115; Libutz and Prihoda (1984); Long et al. (1984); McCall (1984); Riley et al., (1987), pp. 233, 240; and Scitovsky (1984).

4. The *delayed degenerative* label is from Olshansky and Ault (1987). Fuchs (1984a), p. 147, computes the increase in average life expectancy for a sixty-five-year-old as 4.5 years in just the fifteen years from 1965 to 1980. Fries, who pioneered the "compression of morbidity"/"squaring of the curve" thesis (1980), admits some of the contrary evidence but still produces interesting data that preventive care is postponing morbidity faster than it is lengthening life (1988).

5. For the following figures and qualifications, see Scitovsky (1984).

6. Aaron and Schwartz (1984), p. 96. See Singer et al. (1983) for evidence that shifting patients from intensive to nonintensive care need not increase mortality.

202   STRONG MEDICINE

7. Mor and Kidder (1985), p. 414.

8. For expressions along these lines, see Blumenthal, Schlesinger, and Drumheller (1986), p. 723; Siegler (1984), p. 27; and Bayer et al. (1983), p. 1492. In various public and academic forums I have repeatedly heard this sort of view expressed, sometimes by professional ethicists.

9. *Republic,* III, 406C, as cited in Battin (1987), p. 70.

10. *The Twilight of the Idols,* p. 36, as cited in Battin (1987), p. 70.

11. Among others in this long line of cases, see *In the Matter of Karen Quinlan,* 70 N.J. Reports 10 (1976); and *In the Matter of the Welfare of Bertha Colyer,* 220 P. 2d 738 (1983).

12. For these and other considerations that mark off duty from virtue, see Reeder (1982) and Peters (1986b). I am assuming here that the effects on others are not intrusions on their rights. On the troublesome threat of virtues shifting over too easily into duties, see Kagan (1984); and in a related though more legal-duty context, Lipkin (1983) and Weinrib (1980).

13. Callahan (1987), pp. 25–51; and Hardwig (1988).

14. Barrington (1980), p. 97. Battin (1987) introduced me to this quotation.

15. Eys and Vaux (1985).

16. Veatch (1988a), p. 35.

17. Veatch (1988a), p. 39.

18. Beside Veatch, another example of misplaced worry is Battin (1987). Battin argues that people in an "original position" would agree to a future moral system in which suicide was socially encouraged for people with seriously debilitating, chronic diseases of old age. As Wikler (1987), p. 96, points out, the persuasiveness of her argument depends repeatedly on the assumption that the major alternative to such encouraged suicide—rationing care for the very elderly—will inevitably deny even palliative care.

19. Wikler (1988), p. 66.

20. Wikler (1988), p. 62.

21. This is almost—though, with the emphasis on cost-benefit ratios, not quite—the key point about the need for a more time-neutral, comprehensive, lifetime allocation perspective made by Daniels (1988), pp. 57–63.

22. Veatch (1988a), p. 40.

23. Prottas, Segal, and Sapolsky (1983); and Moskop (1987b), p. 43. See also Moskof (1987a).

24. One of the sharpest and perhaps most telling criticisms of the British denial of dialysis in older age is its disguised, hidden character. See Francis and Francis (1987) and Winslow (1986). The Francises criticize both the absence of decision-making participation by those affected and the NHS's failure to acknowledge to the public that real rationing is even the issue, pretending only that care of "no significant value" is being denied. I am not sure that their first charge is correct. In the context of a national health service, would we expect the direct prior participation of these patients in the formation of this policy? The second count may appear more clearly telling, but even here it might be that we have misunderstood the larger British situation. The NHS has never adopted a national policy of denying care to older dialysis patients. Their cost-benefit assessments of dialysis overall have undoubtedly led them to see it as a truly borderline case for what the system can afford if other good things are already shut out. Regional authorities then understandably decide to keep the supply of dialysis facilities distinctly short, and consequently individual physicians aware of that scarcity end up rationing out the older patients as the least objectionable choice. I am quite sure there is a problem here with what patients are then told—"There's nothing much we can do for you," and so on—but I am not sure the policymaking process here is terribly deficient.

25. Neu and Kjellstrand (1986), p. 17, note that one of six patients older than sixty appear to voluntarily withdraw themselves from dialysis.

26. A suggestion by Fries (1988), p. 412, though he leaves it undefended.

27. The case for saying this about really severe dementia is put persuasively by Brock (1988), especially pp. 89–91. See also the related wealth of points by Buchanan (1988), especially p. 299. These two pieces are expanded in a forthcoming volume by Brock and Buchanan, *Deciding for Others: The Ethics of Surrogate Decision-Making* (Cambridge University Press).

28. Concerning long-term care, see the comprehensive assessments and proposals by Somers (1982) and Gillick (1984).

References

Aaron, Henry J., and William B. Schwartz, 1984. *The Painful Prescription: Rationing Hospital Care.* Washington, D.C.: Brookings Institution.

Ackerman, Bruce A. 1985. "Talking and Trading." *Columbia Law Review* 85 (June): 899–904.

Agich, George J. 1985. "Daniels on the Basic Minimum of Health Care?" Paper presented at the American Philosophical Association meetings, Western Division, 1985.

Agich, George J., and Charles E., Begley, eds. 1986. *The Price of Health: Cost-Benefit Analysis and Efficiency in Medicine.* Dordrecht, Neth.: D. Reidel.

Alchian, Armen A., ed., 1973. *The Economics of Charity: Essays on the Comparative Economics and Ethics of Giving and Selling, with Applications to Blood.* London: Institute of Economic Affairs.

American Jurisprudence, 2d series 1977. *Proof of Facts.* Rochester: Lawyers Cooperative.

American Medical Association Board of Trustees. 1986. "Media Advertising for Tobacco Products." *Journal of the American Medical Association* 255 (February 28): 1033.

———. 1987. "Report of the Special Task Force on Professional Liability and Insurance and the Advisory Panel on Professional Liability." *Journal of the American Medical Association* 257 (February 13): 810–12.

American Medical Association Special Task Force on Professional Liability and Insurance. 1984. *Professional Liability in the '80s. Report I and Report II.* Chicago: American Medical Association.

Anderson, Elizabeth. 1988. "Values, Risks, and Market Norms." *Philosophy and Public Affairs* 17 (Winter): 54–65.

Andrews, Lori B. 1986. "My Body, My Property." *Hastings Center Report* 16 (October): 28–38.

Angell, Marcia. 1985. "Cost Containment and the Physician." *Journal of the American Medical Association* 254 (September 6): 1203–7.

Annas, George J. 1984. "Life, Liberty, and the Pursuit of Organ Sales." *Hastings Center Report* 14 (February): 22–23.

———. 1985. "No Cheers for Temporary Artificial Hearts." *Hastings Center Report* 15 (October): 27–28.

Arbogast, Rebecca. 1986. "A Proposal to Regulate the Manner of Tobacco Advertising." *Journal of Health Politics, Policy and Law* 11 (Fall): 393–420.

Arneson, Richard. 1982. "The Principle of Fairness and Free-Rider Problems." *Ethics* 92 (April): 616–33.

Atiyah, P. S. 1982. "A Legal Perspective on Recent Contributions to the Valuation of Life." In Jones-Lee, ed., pp. 185–201.

———. 1986. "Medical Malpractice and the Contract/Tort Boundary." *Law and Contemporary Problems* 49 (Spring): 287–304.

Atkinson, A. B., and Joy L. Townsend 1977. "Economic Aspects of Reduced Smoking." *Lancet,* September 3, pp. 492–95.

Audi, Robert. 1986. "Cost-Benefit Analysis, Monetary Value, and Medical Decision." In Agich and Begley, eds., pp. 113–31.

Avorn, Jerry. 1984. "Benefit and Cost Analysis in Geriatric Care: Turning Age Discrimination into Health Policy." *New England Journal of Medicine* 310 (May 17): 1294–1301.

Bailey, Martin J. 1980. *Reducing Risks to Life: Measurement of the Benefits.* Washington, D.C.: American Enterprise Institute.

Baily, Mary Ann. 1985. "Introduction." In Baily and Cikins, eds., pp. 1–10.

———. 1986. "Rationing Medical Care: Processes for Defining Adequacy." In Agich and Begley, eds., pp. 165–84.

Baily, Mary Ann, and Warren Cikins, eds. 1985. *The Effects of Litigation on Health Care Costs.* Washington, D.C.: Brookings Institution.

Baldwin, John C. 1988. "Lung Transplantation." *Journal of the American Medical Association* 259 (April 15): 2286–87.

Barrington, Mary Rose. 1980. "Apologia for Suicide." In Battin and Mayo, eds., pp. 90–103.

Bassoli, Gloria J. 1986. "Health Care for the Indigent: Overview of Critical Issues." *Health Services Research* 21 (August): 353–93.

Battin, Margaret P. 1987. "Age-Rationing and the Just Distribution of Health Care: Is There a Duty to Die?" In Smeeding, ed., pp. 69–94.

Battin, Margaret P., and David J. Mayo, eds. 1980. *Suicide: The Philosophical Issues.* New York: St. Martin's Press.

Bayer, Ronald, et al. 1983. "The Care of the Terminally Ill: Morality and Economics." *New England Journal of Medicine* 309 (December 15): 1490–94.

Bayles, Michael D. 1987. *Principles of Law: A Normative Analysis.* Dordrecht, Neth.: D. Reidel.

Becker, Gary S., and George J. Stigler. 1977. "De Gustibus Non Est Disputandum." *American Economic Review* 67 (March): 76–90.

Bell, David E. 1982. "Regret in Decision Making under Uncertainty." *Operations Research* 30 (September–October): 961–81.

Bell, Nora K., and Barry M. Loewer. 1985. "What Is Wrong with 'Wrongful Life' Cases?" *Journal of Medicine and Philosophy* 10 (May): 127–45.

Bennett, Jonathan. 1985. "Morality and Consequences." In Sterba, ed., pp. 23–29.

Berry, Ralph E., Jr., and Joseph P. Boland. 1977. *The Economic Cost of Alcohol Abuse.* New York: Free Press.

Blendon, Robert J., et al. 1986. "Uncompensated Care by Hospitals or Public Insurance for the Poor: Does It Make a Difference?" *New England Journal of Medicine* 314 (May 1): 1160–63.

Blodgett, N. 1985. "Hedonic Damages." *American Bar Association Journal* 71 (January): 25–52.

Blohme, I., H. Gabel, and H. Brynger. 1981. "The Living Donor in Renal Transplantation." *Scandinavian Journal of Urology and Nephrology* 64 (Supplement): 143–51.

Blomquist, Glenn. 1982. "Estimating the Value of Life and Safety: Recent Developments." In Jones-Lee, ed., pp. 27–40.

Blumenthal, David, Mark Schlesinger, and Pamela B. Drumheller. 1986. "The Future of Medicare." *New England Journal of Medicine* 314 (March 13): 722–28.

Blumstein, James F. 1981. "Rationing Medical Resources: A Constitutional, Legal, and Policy Analysis." *Texas Law Review* 59 (November): 1345–1400.

Bohlen, F. 1906. "Voluntary Risk Assumption." *Harvard Law Review* 20 (April): 14–91.

Borna, Shaheen, and Krishna Mantripragada. 1987. "Bartering: An Alternative Policy for Obtaining Human Organs for Transplantation." *Journal of Health Care Marketing* 7 (March): 47–53.

Boyle, Michael H., et al. 1983. "Economic Evaluation of Neonatal Intensive Care of Very-Low-Birth-Weight Infants." *New England Journal of Medicine* 308 (June 2): 1330–37.

Brams, Marion. 1977. "Transplantable Human Organs: Should Their Sale Be Authorized by State Statutes?" *American Journal of Law and Medicine* 3 (Summer) 183–95.

Brandon, William P. 1982. "Health-Related Tax Subsidies." *New England Journal of Medicine* 307 (October 7): 947–50.

British Medical Association. 1980. *The Handbook of Medical Ethics.* London: British Medical Association.

Brock, Daniel W. 1986a. "Commentary: Implications of New Physician Payment Methods for Access to Health Care and Physician Fidelity to Patients' Interests." *Case Western Reserve Law Review* 36 (Summer): 760–70.

———. 1986b. "The Value of Prolonging Human Life." *Philosophical Studies* 50 (November): 401–28.

———. 1988. "Justice and the Severely Demented." *Journal of Medicine and Philosophy* 13: (February): 73–100.

Brock, Daniel W., and Allen E. Buchanan. 1985. "Ethical Issues in For-Profit Health Care." In Gray, ed., pp. 224–49.

Brody, Baruch A. 1981. "Health Care for the Haves and Have Nots: Toward a Just Basis of Distribution." In Shelp, ed., (1981), pp. 151–59.

———. 1983. "Redistribution without Egalitarianism." *Social Philosophy and Policy* 1 (Autumn): 71–87.

Brook, Robert H., and Kathleen N. Lohr. 1986. "Will We Need to Ration Effective Health Care?" *Issues in Science and Technology* 3 (Fall): 68–77.

Broome, John. 1978. "Trying to Value a Life." *Journal of Public Economics* 9 (Winter): 91–100.

———. 1982. "Uncertainty in Welfare Economics, and the Value of Life." In Jones-Lee, ed., pp. 201–17.

Brown, Charles. 1980. "Equalizing Differences in the Labor Market." *Quarterly Journal of Economics* 94 (February): 113–34.

Brown, M. S., and D. Nelkin. 1984. *Workers at Risk: Voices from the Workplace.* Chicago: University of Chicago Press.

Broyer, M. 1982. "Legislation on Organ Donation—The French Experience." *Singapore Medical Journal* 23 (December): 341–43.

Brueckner, Anthony L., and John Martin Fischer. 1986. "Why Is Death Bad?" *Philosophical Studies* 50 (September): 213–221.

Buchanan, Allen E. 1984. "The Right to a Decent Minimum of Health Care." *Philosophy and Public Affairs* 13 (Winter): 55–78.

———. 1985. "Competition, Charity, and the Right to Health Care." Tucson: Department of Philosophy, University of Arizona (unpublished manuscript).

———. 1987. "Justice and Charity." *Ethics* 97 (April): 558–75.

———. 1988. "Advance Directives and the Personal Identity Problem." *Philosophy and Public Affairs* 17 (Fall): 277–302.

Budetti, P., et al. 1980. *The Cost Effectiveness of Neonatal Intensive Care.* Washington, D.C.: Office of Technology Assessment.

Bulger, Roger, J. 1973. *Hippocrates Revisited: A Search for Meaning.* New York: Medcom Press.

Burroughs, John T., and Carl R. Edenhofer, Jr. 1983. "Product Liability Actions in Medical Negligence." *Journal of Legal Medicine* 4 (June): 201–29.

Butler, Michael J. 1985. "The Law of Human Organ Procurement: A Modest Proposal." *Journal of Contemporary Health Law and Policy* 1 (Spring): 195–206.

Butler, Stuart M. 1980. "The Competitive Prescription for Health Costs Inflation." *Backgrounder* (Heritage Foundation) 111 (February 25): 1–24.

Butterfield, L. Joseph. 1981. "Evaluation and Economic Exigency in the NICU." *New England Journal of Medicine* 305 (August 27): 518–19.

Calabresi, Guido. 1985. *Ideals, Beliefs, Attitudes, and the Law: Private Law Perspectives on a Public Law Problem.* Syracuse: Syracuse University Press.

Calabresi, Guido, and Jon T. Hirschoff. 1972. "Toward a Test for Strict Liability in Torts." *Yale Law Journal* 81 (May): 1055–85.

Callahan, Daniel. 1987. *Setting Limits: Medical Goals in an Aging Society.* New York: Simon and Schuster.

Cantaluppi, A., A. Scalamogna, and C. Ponticelli. 1984. "Legal Aspects of Organ Procurement in Different Countries." *Transplantation Proceedings* 16 (February): 102–4.

Caplan, Arthur L. 1983. "Organ Transplants: The Costs of Success." *Hastings Center Report* 13 (December): 23–32.

———. 1984. "Ethical and Policy Issues in the Procurement of Cadaver Organs for Transplantation." *New England Journal of Medicine* 311 (October 11): 981–1033.

———. 1988. "Professional Arrogance and Public Misunderstanding." *Hastings Center Report* 18 (April–May): 34–37.

Capron, Alexander Morgan. 1979. "The Continuing Wrong of 'Wrongful Life.'" In Milunsky and Annas, eds., pp. 81–96.

Cassel, Christine K. 1985. "Doctors and Allocation Decisions: A New Role in the New Medicare." *Journal of Health Politics, Policy, and Law* 10 (Fall): 549–64.

Chambers, Marcia. 1986. "Tough Transplant Questions Raised by 'Baby Jesse' Case." *New York Times,* June 15, pp. A1, A12.

Chase, Samuel B., Jr., ed. 1968. *Problems in Public Expenditure Analysis.* Washington, D.C.: Brookings Institution.

Childress, James F. 1987. "Some Moral Connections between Organ Procurement and Organ Distribution." *Journal of Contemporary Health Law and Policy* 3 (Spring): 85–110.

Churchill, David N., Janet Morgan, and George W. Torrance. 1984. "Quality of Life in End-Stage Renal Disease." *Peritoneal Dialysis Bulletin* 4 (January–March): 20–23.

Churchill, Larry R. 1987. *Rationing Health Care in America: Perceptions and Principles of Justice.* Notre Dame, Ind.: University of Notre Dame Press.

Coleman, Jules. 1980. "Efficiency, Utility, and Wealth Maximization." *Hofstra Law Review* 8 (Spring): 509.

Coleman, Jules, and Jeffrey Murphy. 1985. *Philosophy of Law.* Belmont, Calif.: Wadsworth.

Conklin, Thomas W. 1984. "Wrongful Death Damages: Expansion, Inflation, Discounts, and Taxes—The Numbers Game." *Trial Lawyers Guide* 28 (Fall): 249–96.

Cook, Philip J., and Daniel A. Graham. 1977. "The Demand for Insurance and Protection: The Case of Irreplaceable Commodities." *Quarterly Journal of Economics* 91 (February): 143–56.

Cowan, Dale H., et al. 1987. *Human Organ Transplantation: Societal, Medical-Legal, Regulatory, and Reimbursement Issues.* Ann Arbor, Mich.: Health Administration Press.

Culyer, Anthony J. 1976. *Need and the National Health Service.* London: Martin Robertson.

———. 1977 "Blood and Altruism: An Economic Review." In Johnson, ed., pp. 39–58.

———. 1978. "Need, Values and Health Status Measurement." In Culyer and Wright, eds., pp. 9–31.

———. 1985. "Health Service Efficiency—Appraising the Appraisers." Centre for Health Economics, University of York, (U.K.), Discussion Paper no. 10.

Culyer, Anthony J., and John Posnett. 1985. "Would You Choose the Welfare State?" *Economic Affairs* 5 (January–March): 40–42.

Culyer, Anthony J., and K. G. Wright, eds. 1978. *Economic Aspects of Health Services.* London: Martin Robertson.

Culyer, Anthony J., Alan Maynard, and Alan Williams. 1981. "Alternative Systems of Health Care Provision: An Essay on Motes and Beams." In Olson, ed., pp. 131–50.

Curran, William J. 1985. "Economic and Legal Considerations in Emergency Care." *New England Journal of Medicine* 312 (February 7): 374–75.

Daniels, Norman. 1982. "Am I My Parents' Keeper?" *Midwest Studies in Philosophy* 7: 517–40.

———. 1985a *Just Health Care.* Cambridge: Cambridge University Press.

———. 1985b. "Fair Equality of Opportunity and Decent Minimums: A Reply to Buchanan." *Philosophy and Public Affairs* 14 (Winter): 106–10.

——. 1986. "Why Saying No to Patients in the United States Is So Hard." *New England Journal of Medicine* 314 (May 22): 1381–83.

——. 1988. *Am I My Parents' Keeper? An Essay on Justice between the Young and the Old.* New York: Oxford University Press.

Danzon, Patricia M. 1985a. *Medical Malpractice: Theory, Evidence, and Public Policy.* Cambridge, Mass.: Harvard University Press.

——. 1985b. "The Medical Malpractice System: Facts and Reforms." In Baily and Cikins, eds., pp. 28–35.

Department of Health and Social Security (U.K.). 1972. *Smoking and Health: A Study of the Effects of a Reduction in Cigarette Smoking on Mortality and Morbidity Rates, on Health Care and Social Security Expenditure and on Productive Potential.* London: Department of Health and Social Security.

Dickens, Bernard M. 1977. "The Control of Living Body Materials." *University of Toronto Law Journal* 27 (Winter): 142–98.

DiFranza, Joseph R., et al. 1987. "Legislative Efforts to Protect Children from Tobacco." *Journal of the American Medical Association* 257 (June 26): 3387–89.

Dougherty, Charles J. 1987. "Body Futures: The Case against Margeting Organs." *Health Progress* 68 (June): 51–55.

Dowie, Jack, 1982. "Comments on 'A Legal Perspective on Recent Contributions to the Valuation of Life.'" In Jones-Lee, ed., pp. 265–71.

Drake, Alvin M., Stan N. Finkelstein, and Harvey M. Sapolsky. 1982. *The American Blood Supply.* Cambridge, Mass.: MIT Press.

Dukeminier, Jesse. 1970. "Supplying Organs for Transplantation." *Michigan Law Review* 68 (April): 811–66.

Dunham, Andrew, James A. Morone, and William White. 1982. "Restoring Medical Markets: Implications for the Poor." *Journal of Health Politics, Policy and Law* 7 (Summer): 488–500.

Dworkin, Ronald M. 1980. "Is Wealth a Value?" *Journal of Legal Studies* 9 (March): 191–226.

——. 1981. "What Is Equality? Part 1: Equality of Welfare" and "What Is Equality? Part 2: Equality of Resources." *Philosophy and Public Affairs* 10 (Summer and Fall): 185–246, 283–345.

——. 1986a. "Autonomy and the Demented Self." *Milbank Quarterly* 64 (Supplement 2) 4–16.

——. 1986b. *Law's Empire.* Cambridge, Mass.: Harvard University Press.

Dyer, Allen R. 1986. "Patients, Not Costs, Come First." *Hastings Center Report* 16 (February): 5–7.

Eggers, Paul W. 1988. "Effect of Transplantation on the Medicare End-Stage Renal Disease Program." *New England Journal of Medicine* 318 (January 28): 223–29.

Eliahou, H. 1982. "Dialysis and Transplantation in Israel—An Overview." *Singapore Medical Journal* 23 (December): 338–40.

Ellin, Joseph. 1988. "Potentiality and Rights." *Newsletter on Philosophy and Medicine* [American Philosophical Association] (March): 3–4.

Engelhardt, H. Tristram, Jr. 1975. "Case Studies in Bioethics: A Demand to Die." *Hastings Center Report* 5 (June): 10–11.

——. 1984. "Allocating Scarce Medical Resources and the Availability of Organ Transplantation." *New England Journal of Medicine* 311 (July 5): 66–71.

———. 1986. *The Foundations of Bioethics.* New York: Oxford University Press.

Enthoven, Alain C. 1978. "Consumer Choice Health Plan." *New England Journal of Medicine* 298 (March 23 and 30): 650–58, 709–20.

Epstein, Richard A. 1976. "Medical Malpractice: The Case for Contract." *American Bar Foundation Research Journal* 76: 87–149.

———. 1980. *A Theory of Strict Liability: Toward a Reformulation of Tort Law.* San Francisco: Cato Institute.

———. 1986. "Medical Malpractice, Imperfect Information, and the Contractual Foundation for Medical Services." *Law and Contemporary Problems* 49 (Spring): 201–12.

Evans, Roger W., et al. 1985. "The Quality of Life of Patients with End-Stage Renal Disease." *New England Journal of Medicine* 312 (February 28): 553–59.

Eys, Jan Van, and Kenneth Vaux. 1985. "A Declaration of Faith and Health." *Christian Century,* July 3–10, pp. 643–45.

Farfor, J. A. 1977. "Organs for Transplant: Courageous Legislation." *British Medical Journal,* February 19, pp. 497–98.

Farley, Pamela J. 1985. "Who Are the Underinsured?" *Milbank Memorial Fund Quarterly* 63: 476–503.

Fein, Rashi. 1986. *Medical Care, Medical Costs.* Cambridge, Mass.: Harvard University Press.

Feinberg, Joel. 1984. *The Moral Limits of the Criminal Law. Vol. I: Harm to Others.* New York: Oxford University Press.

———. 1986. "Wrongful Life and the Counterfactual Element in Harming." *Social Philosophy and Policy* 4 (Autumn): 145–78.

Fischer, Allen, and David K. Stevenson. 1987. "The Consequences of Uncertainty: An Empirical Approach to Medical Decision Making in Neonatal Intensive Care." *Journal of the American Medical Association* 258 (October 9): 1929–31.

Fischer, John Martin, and Robert H. Ennis. 1986. "Causation and Liability." *Philosophy and Public Affairs* 15 (Winter): 33–40.

Fleck, Leonard M. 1987. "The Physician and the Rationing of Health Care Resources." *Newsletter on Philosophy and Medicine* [American Philosophical Association] (Summer): 1–3.

Fortess, Eric E., and Marshall B. Kapp. 1985. "Medical Uncertainty, Diagnostic Testing, and Legal Liability." *Law, Medicine and Health Care* 13 (October): 213–18.

Francis, John G., and Leslie P. Francis. "Rationing of Health Care in Britain: An Ethical Critique of Public Policy-Making." In Smeeding, ed., pp. 119–34.

Frank, Robert H. 1982. "Envy and the Optimal Purchase of Unobservable Commodities: The Case of Safety." In Jones-Lee, ed., pp. 145–57.

Frech, H. E. III, ed. 1988. *Health Care in America: The Political Economy of Hospitals and Health Insurance.* San Francisco: Pacific Research Institute for Public Policy.

Freeman, John M. 1984. "Early Management and Decision Making for the Treatment of Myelomeningocele: A Critique." *Pediatrics* 73 (April): 564–65.

Fried, Charles. 1981. *Contract as Promise.* Cambridge, Mass.: Harvard University Press.

Friedman, David D. 1986. "Comments on 'Rationing and Publicity.'" In Agich and Begley, eds., pp. 217–24.

Friedman, Emily. 1984. "Can 'Essential Services' Be Defined?" *Hospitals* 58 (November 1): 105–8.

Fries, James F. 1980. "Aging, Natural Death, and the Compression of Morbidity." *New England Journal of Medicine* 303 (July 17): 130–36.

Fries, James F. 1988. "Aging, Illness, and Health Policy: Implications of the Compression of Morbidity." *Perspectives in Biology and Medicine* 31 (Spring): 407–28.

Fuchs, Victor R. 1984a. "'Though Much Is Taken': Reflections on Aging, Health, and Medical Care." *Milbank Memorial Fund Quarterly* 62 (Spring): 143–65.

———. 1984b. "The 'Rationing' of Medical Care." *New England Journal of Medicine* 311 (December 13): 1572–73.

Gallo, Nick. 1986. "Insurance Costs: Main Event for the Fat Cats." *Weekly* [Seattle, Wa.], January 8–14, pp. 16–17.

Ghosh, D., D. Lees, and W. Seal. 1975. "Optimal Motorway Speed and Some Valuations of Time and Life." *Manchester School of Economic and Social Studies* 43 (June): 134–43.

Gibson, Mary. 1985. "Consent and Autonomy." In Gibson, ed., pp. 141–168.

Gibson, Mary, ed. 1985. *To Breathe Freely: Risk, Consent, and Air.* Totowa, N.J.: Rowman and Allanheld.

Gilbert, Neil. 1983. *Capitalism and the Welfare State: Dilemmas of Social Benevolence.* New Haven: Yale University Press.

Gillick, Muriel R. 1984. "Is the Care of the Chronically Ill a Medical Prerogative?" *New England Journal of Medicine* 310 (January 19): 190–93.

Ginsburg, Paul B., and Frank A. Sloan. 1984. "Hospital Cost-Shifting." *New England Journal of Medicine* 310 (April 5): 893–98.

Ginzburg, Eli. 1987. "A Hard Look at Cost Containment." *New England Journal of Medicine* 316 (April 30): 1151–54.

Godfrey, Christine, and Melanie Powell. 1986a. "Addiction and Health Information: Central Concepts Linking Estimates of Alcohol Costs with Prevention Policy." ESRC Addiction Research Centre, Centre for Health Economics, University of York (U.K.) (unpublished).

———. 1986b. "The Confusion of Economic Costs: Estimates of the Cost of Alcohol and Tobacco Consumption and Their Relation to Government Preventive Health Policy." ESRC Addiction Research Centre, Centre for Health Economics, University of York (U.K.) (unpublished).

Gorovitz, Samuel. 1984. "Against Selling Bodily Parts." *QQ: Report from the Center for Philosophy and Public Policy* 4 (Spring): 9–12.

Graham, Clay P. 1984. "Helmetless Motorcyclists—Easy Riders Facing Hard Facts: The Rise of the 'Motorcycle Helmet Defense'" *Ohio State Law Journal* 41 (April): 233–69.

Graham, Gordon. 1987. "The Doctor, the Rich, and the Indigent." *Journal of Medicine and Philosophy* 12 (February): 51–62.

Graham, Julie, and Dan M. Shakow. 1981. "Risk and Reward: Hazard Pay for Workers." *Environment* 23 (October): 14–20, 44.

Graham, Julie, Dan M. Shakow, and Christopher Cyr. 1983. "Risk Compensation—Theory and Practice." *Environment* 25 (January–February): 14–40.

Gray, Bradford H., ed. 1985. *The New Health Care for Profit: Doctors and Hospitals in a Competitive Environment.* Washington, D.C.: National Academy Press.

Green, David G. 1986. *Challenge to the NHS: A Study of Competition in American Health Care and the Lessons for Britain.* London: Institute for Economic Affairs.

Gross, R. H., et al. 1983. "Early Management and Decision Making for the Treatment of Myelomeningocele." *Pediatrics* 72: 450–55.

Gudex, Claire. 1986. "QALYs and Their Use by the Health Service." York, U.K.: University of York, Centre for Health Economics, Discussion Paper 20.

Hadley, Jack, 1982. *More Medical Care, Better Health?* Washington, D.C.: Urban Institute Press.

Hagard, S., F. Carter, and R. G. Milne. 1976. "Screening for Spina Bifida Cystica: A Cost-Benefit Analysis." *British Journal of Preventive and Social Medicine* 30 (January): 40–53.

Hagen, Piet J. 1982. *Blood: Gift or Merchandise.* New York: Alan Liss.

Halper, Thomas. 1985. "Life and Death in a Welfare State: End-Stage Renal Disease in the United Kingdom." *Milbank Memorial Fund Quarterly* 63 (Winter): 52–93.

Hardwig, John. 1988. "Donating Your Health Care Benefits." *Hastings Center Report* 18: (April): 8–9.

Harris, John. 1975. "The Survival Lottery." *Philosophy* 50 (January): 81–87.

———. 1985. *The Value of Life: An Introduction to Medical Ethics.* London: Routledge and Kegan Paul.

———. 1986. "QALYfying the Value of Life" (revised version of address to British Medical Association Annual Scientific Meeting, Oxford, April 1986). University of Manchester (U.K.), Department of Education (manuscript).

Hastings Center. 1987. "Imperiled Newborns." *Hastings Center Report* 17 (December): 5–32.

Havighurst, Clark C. 1986. "Altering the Applicable Standard of Care." *Law and Contemporary Problems* 49 (Spring): 265–76.

Hodgson, Thomas A. 1983. "The State of the Art of Cost-of-Illness Estimates." *Advances in Health Economics and Health Services Research* 4: 129–64.

Hoffman, W. S. 1985. "Price Discrimination in Medicine." *Hastings Center Report* 15 (October): 19–20.

Holder, Angela. 1981. "Is Existence Ever An Injury? The Wrongful Life Cases." In Spicker, Healey, and Engelhardt, eds., pp. 225–39.

Hollis, Martin. 1983. "Rational Preferences." *Philosophical Forum* 14 (Spring–Summer): 246–62.

Hubbell, F., et al. 1985. "The Impact of Routine Admission Chest X-ray Films on Patient Care." *New England Journal of Medicine* 312 (January 24): 209–13.

Hyman, M. M. 1981. "Cirrhosis Deaths in the U.S. and Massachusetts." *Journal of Studies on Alcohol* 42 (March): 336–43.

Iglehart, John K. 1983. "Transplantation: The Problem of Limited Resources." *New England Journal of Medicine* 309 (July 14): 123–28.

———. 1985. "Medical Care of the Poor—A Growing Problem." *New England Journal of Medicine* 313 (July 4): 59–63.

Ireland, Marilyn J. 1973. "The Legal Framework of the Market for Blood." In Alchian, ed., pp. 173–78.

James, Fleming, Jr. 1968. "Assumption of Risk: Unhappy Reincarnation." *Yale Law Journal* 78 (December): 185–97.

James, Mary. 1988. "The Organ Transplant Catalog." *Hippocrates* 2 (May–June): 46.

Joe, Thomas C. W., Judith Meltzer, and Peter Yu. 1985. "Arbitrary Access to Care: The Case for Reforming Medicaid." *Health Affairs* 4 (Spring): 59–73.

Johnson, David B., ed. 1977. *Blood Policy: Issues and Alternatives.* Washington, D.C.: American Enterprise Institute.

Jones-Lee, M. W. 1974. "The Value of Changes in the Probability of Death or Injury." *Journal of Political Economy* 82 (July–August): 835–49.

Jones-Lee, M. W., ed. 1982. *The Value of Life and Safety.* Leiden, Neth.: North-Holland.

Jonsen, Albert, R. 1985. "Organ Transplants and the Principle of Fairness." *Law, Medicine and Health Care* 13 (February): 37–39, 44.

Kagan, Shelly. 1984. "Does Consequentialism Demand Too Much? Recent Work on the Limits of Obligation." *Philosophy and Public Affairs* 13: (Summer): 239–54.

Kahneman, Daniel, and Amos Tversky. 1979. "Prospect Theory: An Analysis of Decision under Risk." *Econometrica* 47 (March): 263–91.

———. 1982. "The Psychology of Preferences." *Scientific American,* Janaury, pp. 160–73.

Kahneman, Daniel, Paul Slovic, and Amos Tversky, eds. 1982. *Judgment under Uncertainty: Heuristics and Biases.* Cambridge: Cambridge University Press.

Kaplan, Robert M., and James W. Bush. 1982. "Health-Related Quality of Life Measurement for Evaluation Research and Policy Analysis." *Health Psychology* 1 (January): 61–80.

Kass, Leon R. 1985a. "Thinking about the Body." *Hastings Center Report* 15 (February): 20–30.

———. *Toward a More Natural Science: Biology and Human Affairs.* New York: Free Press.

Kelman, Steven. 1984. *What Price Incentives: Economists and the Environment.* Boston: Auburn House.

———. 1986. "A Case for In-Kind Transfers." *Economics and Philosophy* 2 (April): 55–73.

Kennedy, Duncan. 1981. "Cost-Benefit Analysis of Entitlement Problems: A Critique." *Stanford Law Review* 33 (February): 387–445.

Kennedy, Ian. 1979. "The Donation and Transplantation of Kidneys: Should the Law Be Changed." *Journal of Medical Ethics* 5 (January): 13–21.

Kessel, Reuben A. 1958. "Price Discrimination in Medicine." *Journal of Law and Economics* 1 (April): 20–53.

———. 1974. "Tranfused Blood, Serum Hepatitis, and the Coase Theorem." *Journal of Law and Economics* 17 (October): 265–90.

Kind, Paul, Rachel Rosser, and Alan Williams. 1982. "Valuation of Quality of Life: Some Psychometric Evidence." In Jones-Lee, ed., pp. 159–70.

Kinzer, David. 1988. "The Decline and Fall of Deregulation." *New England Journal of Medicine* 318 (January 14): 112–16.

Kitzhaber, John. 1988. "Uncompensated Care—The Threat and the Challenge." *Western Journal of Medicine* 148 (June): 711–16.

Klosko, George. 1987. "Presumptive Benefit, Fairness, and Political Obligation." *Philosophy and Public Affairs* 16 (Summer): 241–59.

Kovar, Mary Grace. 1986. "Expenditures for the Medical Care of Elderly People Living in the Community in 1980." *Milbank Quarterly* 64 (Winter): 100–132.

Krakauer, H., et al. 1983. "The Recent U.S. Experience in the Treatment of End-Stage Renal Disease by Dialysis and Transplantation." *New England Journal of Medicine* 308 (June 23): 1558–63.

Kuhse, Helga, and Peter Singer. 1985. *Should the Baby Live? The Problem of Handicapped Infants.* New York : Oxford University Press.

Lambertson, Mark A. 1984. "Organ Donation Update." *Colorado Lawyer* 13 (April): 615–18.

Lantos, John D., et al. 1988. "Survival after Cardiopulmonary Resuscitation in Babies of Very Low Birth Weight." *New England Journal of Medicine* 318 (January 14): 91–95.

Leichter, Howard. 1981. "Public Policy and the British Experience." *Hastings Center Report* 11 (October): 32–39.

Leonard, Herbert B., and Richard J. Zeckhauser. 1986. "Cost-Benefit Analysis Applied to Risks: Its Philosophy and Legitimacy." In MacLean, ed., pp. 31–48.

Leu, Robert E., and Thomas Schaub. 1983. "Does Smoking Increase Medical Care Expenditure." *Social Science and Medicine* 17: 1907–14.

———. 1985. "More on the Impact of Smoking on Medical Care Expenditures." *Social Science in Medicine* 21 (July) 825–27.

Leventhal, Howard, Kathleen Glynn, and Raymond Fleming. 1987. "Is the Smoking Decision an 'Informed Choice'?" *Journal of the American Medical Association* 257 (June 26): 3373–76.

Levey, Andrew S., Susan Hou, and Harry L. Bush, Jr. 1986. "Kidney Transplantation from Unrelated Living Donors." *New England Journal of Medicine* 314 (April 3): 914–16.

Levi, Isaac. 1986. "The Paradoxes of Allais and Ellsberg." *Economics and Philosophy* 2 (April): 23–53.

Levinsky, Norman G. 1984. "The Doctor's Master." *New England Journal of Medicine* 311 (December 13): 1573–75.

Libutz, J., and R. Prihoda. 1984. "The Use and Costs of Medicare Services in the Last Two Years of Life." *Health Care Financing Review* 5 (Spring): 117–31.

Linnerooth, Joanne. 1982. "Murdering Statistical Lives . . . ?" In Jones-Lee, ed., pp. 229–61.

Lipkin, Robert Justin. 1983. "Beyond Good Samaritans and Moral Monsters: An Individualistic Justification of the General Legal Duty to Rescue." *UCLA Law Review* 31 (October): 252–93.

Lipton, Karen Shoos. 1986. "Blood Donor Services and Liability Issues Relating to Acquired Immune Deficiency Syndrome." *Journal of Legal Medicine* 7 (June): 131–86.

Localio, A. Russell. 1985. "Variations on $962,258: The Misuse of Data on Medical Malpractice." *Law, Medicine and Health Care* 13 (June): 126–27.

Long, Stephen H., et al. 1984. "Medical Expenditures of Terminal Cancer Patients during the Last Year of Life." *Inquiry* 21 (Winter): 315–27.

Loomes, Graham. 1986. "Further Evidence of the Impact of Regret and Disappointment in Choice under Uncertainty." York, U.K.: Institute for Research in the Social Sciences, Discussion Paper 119.

Loomes, Graham, and Robert Sugden. 1982. "Regret Theory: An Alternative Theory of Rationality under Uncertainty." *Economic Journal* 92: (December): 805–24.

———. 1986. "Disappointment and Dynamic Consistency in Choice under Uncertainty." *Review of Economic Studies* 53 (April): 271–82.

Luce, Bryan R., and Stuart O. Schweitzer. 1978. "Smoking and Alcohol Abuse: A Comparison of Their Economic Consequences." *New England Journal of Medicine* 298 (March 9): 569–71.

Luft, Harold S. 1986. "Compensating for Biased Selection in Health Insurance." *Milbank Quarterly* 64 (Fall): 566–91.

McCall, N. 1984. "Utilization and Costs of Medicare Services by Beneficiaries in Their Last Year of Life." *Medical Care* 22 (October): 329–43.

McGarity, Thomas O. 1984. "The New OSHA Rules and the Worker's Right to Know." *Hastings Center Report* 14 (August): 38–45.

McLaughlin, John F., et al. 1985. "Influence of Prognosis on Decisions Regarding the Care of Newborns with Myelodysplasia." *New England Journal of Medicine* 312 (June 20): 1589–94.

MacLean, Douglas. 1986. "Risk and Consent: Philosophical Issues for Centralized Decisions." In MacLean, ed., pp. 17–30.

MacLean, Douglas, ed. 1986. *Values at Risk*. Totowa, N.J.: Rowan and Allanheld.

Mandelblatt, Jeanne S., and Marianne C. Fahs. 1988. "The Cost-Effectiveness of Cervical Cancer Screening for Low-Income Elderly Women." *Journal of the American Medical Association* 259 (April 22–29): 2409–13.

Manga, Pranlal. 1987. "A Commercial Market for Organs? Why Not." *Bioethics* 1 (October): 321–38.

Manninen, Diane L., and Roger W. Evans. 1985. "Public Attitudes and Behavior Regarding Organ Donation." *Journal of the American Medical Association* 253 (June 7): 3111–15.

Markovits, Richard S. 1984. "Duncan's Do Nots: Cost-Benefit Analysis and the Determination of Legal Entitlements." *Stanford Law Review* 36 (May): 1169–98.

Martyn, Susan, Richard Wright, and Leo Clark. 1988. "Required Request for Organ Donation: Moral, Clinical, and Legal Problems." *Hastings Center Report* 18: (April–May): 27–34.

Massachusetts Task Force on Organ Transplantation. 1984. *Report of the Massachusetts Task Force on Organ Transplantation*. Boston: Massachusetts. Department of Public Health.

Matas, Arthur J., et al. 1985. "A Proposal for Cadaver Organ Procurement: Routine Removal with Right of Informed Refusal." *Journal of Health Politics, Policy and Law* 10 (Summer): 231–44.

Mathieu, Deborah, ed. 1988. *Organ Substitution Technology: Ethical, Legal, and Public Policy Issues*. Boulder, Colo.: Westview Press,

May, William F. 1985. "Religious Justifications for Donating Body Parts." *Hastings Center Report* 15 (February): 38–42.

Maynard, Alan, and Anne Ludbrook. 1980. "What's Wrong with the NHS?" *Lloyds Bank Review* 138 (October): 27–41.

Mehlman, Maxwell J. 1986. "Health Care Cost Containment and Medical Technology: A Critique of Waste Theory." *Case Western Reserve Law Review* 36 (Summer): 778–871.

Menzel, Paul T. 1983. *Medical Costs, Moral Choices: A Philosophy of Health Care Economics in America*. New Haven: Yale University Press.

————. 1988. "Scarce Dollars for Saving Lives: The Case of Heart and Liver Transplants." In Mathieu, ed., pp. 155–64.

Meyer, Jack A., with William R. Johnson and Sean Sullivan. 1983. *Passing the Health Care Buck: Who Pays the Hidden Cost?* Washington, D.C.: American Enterprise Institute.

Miller, Frances H. 1985. "Reflections on Organ Transplantation in the United Kingdom." *Law, Medicine and Health Care* 13 (February): 31–32.

Miller, Frances H., and Graham A. H. Miller. 1986. "The Painful Prescription: A Procrustean Perspective." *New England Journal of Medicine* 314 (May 22): 1383–85.

Milunsky, Aubrey, and George J. Annas, eds. 1979. *Genetics and the Law* Vol. II. New York: Plenum Press.

Mishan, Ezra J. 1971. "Evaluation of Life and Limb: A Theoretical Approach." *Journal of Political Economy* 79 (July): 687–706.

————. 1985. "Consistency in the Valuation of Life: A Wild Goose Chase?" In Paul, Miller, and Paul, eds., pp. 152–67.

Mitchell, B. M., and R. J. Vogel. 1975. "Health and Taxes: An Assessment of the Medical Deduction." *Southern Economic Journal* 41 (April): 660–72.

Monheit, Alan C., et al. 1985. "The Employed Uninsured and the Role of Public Policy." *Inquiry* 22 (Winter): 348–64.

Mooney, Gavin. 1986. *Economics, Medicine, and Health Care*. Atlantic Highlands, N.J.: Humanities Press International.

Mor, Vincent, and David Kidder. 1985. "Cost Savings in Hospice: Final Results of the National Hospice Study." *Health Services Research* 20 (October): 407–21.

Morelli, Mario. 1985. "The Fairness Principle." *Philosophy and Law Newsletter* [American Philosophical Association] (Spring): 2–4.

Morreim, E. Haavi. 1985. "The MD and the DRG." *Hastings Center Report* 15 (June): 30–38.

————. 1987a. "Clinicians or Committees—Who Should Cut Costs?" [letter] *Hastings Center Report*. 17 (April): 45.

————. 1987b. "Cost Containment and the Standard of Medical Care." *California Law Review* 75 (October): 1719–63.

————. 1988a. "Cost Constraints as a Malpractice Defense." *Hastings Center Report* 18 (February–March): 5–10.

————. 1988b. Reply to letter. *Hastings Center Report* 18 (April–May): 44.

Mosely, Kathryn L. 1986. "The History of Infanticide in Western Society." *Issues in Law and Medicine* 1 (September) 345–61.

Moskop, John C. 1987a. "The Moral Limits to Federal Funding for Kidney Disease." *Hastings Center Report* 17 (April): 11–15.

————. 1987b. Reply to letters. *Hastings Center Report*. 17 (December): 43–44.

Mulkay, Michael, Trevor Pinch, and Malcolm Ashmore. 1986. "Measuring the Quality of Life: A Sociological Invention Concerning the Application of Economics to Health Care." Department of Sociology, University of York (U.K.) (manuscript).

Murray, Thomas H. 1985. "Why Solutions Continue to Elude Us." *Social Science and Medicine* 20 (November): 1103–8.

————. 1987. "Gifts of the Body and the Needs of Strangers." *Hastings Center Report* 17 (April): 30–38.

Muyskens, James L. 1978. "An Alternative Policy for Obtaining Cadaver Organs for Transplantation." *Philosophy and Public Affairs* 8 (Fall): 88–99.

———. 1987. "Organ Procurement and Allocation Policies: Should Receiving Depend upon Willingness to Give?" Conference paper, Mt. Sinai Hospital, Spring.

Nagel, Thomas. 1985. "Agent-Relative Morality." In Sterba, ed., pp. 15–22.

Neu, Steven, and Carl M. Kjellstrand. 1986. "Stopping Long-Term Dialysis: An Empirical Study of Withdrawal of Life-Supporting Treatment." *New England Journal of Medicine* 314 (January 2): 14–20.

Newacheck, Paul W., et al. 1980. "Income and Illness." *Medical Care* 18 (December): 1165–76.

Nino, C. S. 1983. "A Consensual Theory of Punishment." *Philosophy and Public Affairs* 12 (Fall): 289–306.

Note. 1974. "The Sale of Human Body Parts." *Michigan Law Review* 72 (May): 1182–1264.

Nozick, Robert. 1974. *Anarchy, State, and Utopia.* New York: Basic Books.

Nutter, Donald O. 1987. "Medical Indigency and the Public Health Care Crisis." *New England Journal of Medicine* 316 (April 30): 1156–58.

O'Donnell, Michael. 1986. "One Man's Burden." *British Medical Journal* 293 (July 5): 59.

Ogden, David A. 1983. "Another View on Presumed Consent." *Hastings Center Report* 13 (December): 28.

Olshansky, S. Jay, and Brian A. Ault. 1987. "The Fourth Stage of the Epidemiologic Transition: The Age of Delayed Degenerative Diseases." In Smeeding, ed., pp. 11–43.

Olson, Mancur, ed. 1981. *A New Approach to the Economics of Health Care.* Washington, D.C.: American Enterprise Institute.

Oster, Gerry, Graham A. Colditz, and Nancy L. Kelly. 1984. *The Economic Costs of Smoking and Benefits of Quitting.* Lexington, Mass. D. C. Heath.

Overcast, Thomas D., et al. 1984. "Problems in the Identification of Potential Organ Donors." *Journal of the American Medical Association* 251 (March 23–30): 1560.

Pallis, C. 1982. "The Present Status of Kidney Donation in the United Kingdom." *Singapore Medical Journal* 23 (December): 335–37.

Parfit, Derek. 1984. *Reasons and Persons.* Oxford: Oxford University Press.

Paul, Ellen Frankel, Fred D. Miller, Jr., and Jeffrey Paul, eds. 1985. *Ethics and Economics.* Oxford: Basil Blackwell.

Pauly, Mark V. 1984. "Is Cream-Skimming a Problem for the Competitive Medical Market?" *Journal of Health Economics* 3 (April): 87–95.

———. 1988. "A Primer on Competition in Medical Markets." In Frech, ed., pp. 27–71.

Pellegrino, Edmund D. 1973. "Toward an Expanded Medical Ethics: The Hippocratic Ethic Revisited." In Bulger, ed., pp. 133–47.

Perlman, M., and J. van der Gaag., eds. 1981. *Health, Economics, and Health Economics.* Leiden, Neth.: North-Holland.

Perry, Clifton. 1982. "Wrongful Life and the Comparison of Harms." *Westminster Institute Review* 1 (April): 7–9.

Peters, David A. 1984. "Marketing Organs for Transplantation." *Dialysis and Transplantation* 13 (January): 40–42.

————. 1986a. "Protecting Autonomy in Organ Procurement Procedures: Some Over-looked Issues." *Milbank Quarterly* 64 (Spring): 241–70.

————. 1986b. "Rationales for Organ Donation: Charity or Duty?" *Journal of Medical Humanities and Bioethics* 7 (Fall–Winter): 106–21.

————. 1988. "A Unified Approach to Organ/Tissue Procurement and Distribution." Unpublished paper, Department of Philosophy, University of Wisconsin, River Falls.

Phibbs, Ciaran S., Ronald L. Williams, and Roderic H. Phibbs. 1981. "Newborn Risk Factors and Costs of Neonatal Intensive Care." *Pediatrics* 68 (September): 313–21.

Posner, Richard A. 1977. *Economic Analysis of Law*, 2d ed. New York: Little, Brown.

————. 1980. "The Ethical and Political Basis of the Efficiency Norm in Common Law Adjudication." *Hofstra Law Review* 8: (Spring): 487–509.

President's Commission for the Study of Ethical Problems in Medicine. 1983. *Securing Access to Health Care: The Ethical Implications of Differences in the Availability of Health Services.* Vol. I. Washington, D.C.: U.S. Government Printing Office.

Prosser, William L. 1971. *Handbook of the Law of Torts,* 4th ed. St. Paul: West.

Prottas, Jeffrey M. 1985. "Organ Procurement in Europe and the United States." *Milbank Memorial Fund Quarterly* 63 (Winter) 94–126.

Prottas, Jeffrey, Mark Segal, and Harvey M. Sapolsky. 1983. "Cross-National Differences in Dialysis Rates." *Health Care Financing Review* 4 (Winter) 91–103.

QQ. 1988. "Rethinking Rationality." *QQ: Report from the Institute for Philosophy and Public Policy* 8 (Winter): 1–5.

Rachels, James. 1986. *The End of Life: Euthanasia and Morality.* New York: Oxford University Press.

Ravenholt, R. T. 1985. "Tobacco's Impact on 20th-Century U.S. Mortality Patterns." *American Journal of Preventive Medicine* 1985 (January): 4–17.

Rawls, John. 1971. *A Theory of Justice.* Cambridge, Mass.: Harvard University Press.

Reeder, John P. 1982. "Beneficence, Supererogation, and Role Duty." In Shelp, ed., pp. 83–108.

Regan, Donald H. 1983. "Paternalism, Freedom, Identity, and Commitment." In Sartorius, ed., pp. 113–38.

Reinhardt, Uwe E. 1987. "Resource Allocation in Health Care." *Milbank Quarterly* 65 (Spring): 153–76.

Reynolds, Roger A., John A. Rizzo, and Martin L. Gonzalez. 1987. "The Cost of Medical Professional Liability." *Journal of the American Medical Association.* 257 (May 22–29): 2776–81.

Rice, Dorothy P., et al. 1986. "The Economic Costs of the Health Effects of Smoking, 1984." *Milbank Quarterly* 64 (Fall): 489–547.

Rice, Dorothy P., Thomas A. Hodgson, and Andrea N. Kopstein. 1985. "The Economic Costs of Illness: A Replication and Update." *Health Care Financing Review* 7 (Fall): 61–80.

Richards, Dickinson W. 1973. "Hippocrates and History: The Arrogance of Humanism." In Bulger, ed., pp. 14–29.

Riddiough, Michael A., Jane E. Sisk, and John C. Bell. 1983. "Influenza Vaccination—Cost-Effectiveness and Public Policy." *Journal of the American Medical Association* 249 (June 17): 3189–95.

Riley, Gerald, et al. 1987. "The Use and Costs of Medicare Services by Cause of Death." *Inquiry* 24 (Fall): 233–44.

Robinson, Glen O. 1986. "Rethinking the Allocation of Medical Malpractice Risks between Patients and Providers." *Law and Contemporary Problems* 49 (Spring): 173–200.

Robinson, James C. 1986. "Philosophical Origins of the Economic Valuation of Life."*Milbank Quarterly* 64 (Winter): 133–55.

Robinson, James, and Harold S. Luft. 1987. "Competition and the Cost of Hospital Care, 1972 to 1982." *Journal of the American Medical Association* 257 (June 19): 3241–45.

Rosser, Rachel. 1984. "A History of the Development of Health Indicators." In Smith, ed., pp. 50–62.

Rosser, Rachel, and Paul Kind. 1978. "A Scale of Valuations of States of Illness: Is There a Social Consensus?" *International Journal of Epidemiology* 7 (Fall) 347–58.

Russell, Louise B. 1986. *Is Prevention Better Than Cure?* Washington, D.C.: Brookings Institution.

Sager, Alan. 1988. "Prices of Equitable Access: The New Massachusetts Health Insurance Law." *Hastings Center Report* 18 (June–July): 21–25.

Samuelson, Paul. 1958. "An Exact Consumption-Loan Model of Interest With or Without the Social Contrivance of Money."*Journal of Political Economy* 66 (December): 467–82.

Sapolsky, Harvey M. 1984. Review of Hagen (1982). *Journal of Health Politics, Policy and Law* 8 (Winter): 814–15.

Sartorius, Rolf, ed. 1983. *Paternalism.* Minneapolis: University of Minnesota Press.

Schelling, Thomas C. 1968. "The Life You Save May Be Your Own." In Chase, ed., pp. 127–62.

———. 1984. *Choice and Consequence.* Cambridge, Mass.: Harvard University Press.

———. 1986. "Economics and Cigarettes." *Preventive Medicine* 15 (September): 549–60.

Schiff, Robert L., et al. 1986. "Transfers to a Public Hospital: A Prospective Study of 467 Patients." *New England Journal of Medicine* 314 (February 27): 552–57.

Schwartz, Howard S. 1984. "Bioethical and Legal Considerations in Increasing the Supply of Transplantable Organs: From UAGA to 'Baby Fae.'" *American Journal of Law and Medicine* 10: 397–437.

Schwartz, William B. 1987. "The Inevitable Failure of Current Cost-Containment Strategies: Why they Can Provide Only Temporary Relief." *JAMA* 257 (January 9): 220–24.

Schwartz, William B., and Neil K. Komesar. 1978. "Doctors, Damages and Deterrence: An Economic View of Medical Malpractice." *New England Journal of Medicine* 298 (June 8): 1282–89.

Schwindt, Richard, and Aidan R. Vining. 1986. "Proposal for a Future Delivery Market for Transplant Organs." *Journal of Health Politics, Policy and Law* 11 (Fall): 483–500.

Scitovsky, Anne A. 1984. "'The High Cost of Dying': What Do the Data Show?" *Milbank Memorial Fund Quarterly* 62 (Fall): 591–608.

Scitovsky, Anne A., and Alexander M. Capron. 1986. "Medical Care at the End of Life: The Interaction of Economics and Ethics." *Annual Review of Public Health* 7: 59–75.

Scott, Russell. 1981. *The Body as Property.* New York: Viking Press.

Sen, Amartya. 1983. "Liberty and Social Choice." *Journal of Philosophy* 80 (January): 5–28.

Shannon, Daniel C., et al. 1981. "Survival, Cost of Hospitalization, and Prognosis in Infants Critically Ill with Respiratory Distress Syndrome Requiring Mechanical Ventilation." *Critical Care Medicine* 9 (February): 94–97.

Shelp, Earl E., ed., 1981. *Justice and Health Care.* Dordrecht: D. Reidel.

———. 1982. *Beneficence and Health Care.* Dordrecht: D. Reidel.

Shoven, John B., Jeffrey O. Sundberg, and John P. Bunker. 1987. "The Social Security Cost of Smoking." Cambridge Mass.: National Bureau of Economic Research, Working Paper no. 2234.

Siegler, Mark. 1984. "Should Age Be a Criterion of Health Care?" *Hastings Center Report* 14 (October): 24–27.

Simmons, A. John. 1979. "The Principle of Fair Play." *Philosophy and Public Affairs* 8 (Summer): 307–37.

Sinclair, John C., et al. 1981. "Evaluation of Neonatal-Intensive-Care Programs." *New England Journal of Medicine* 305 (August 27): 489–93.

Singer, Daniel E., et al. 1983. "Rationing Intensive Care—Physician Responses to a Resource Shortage." *New England Journal of Medicine* 309 (November 10): 1155–60.

Slovic, Paul, Baruch Fischoff, and Sarah Lichtenstein. 1982. "Facts versus Fears: Understanding Perceived Risk." In Kahneman, Slovic, and Tversky, eds., pp. 463–89.

Smedley, T. A. 1984. "Some Order Out of Chaos in Wrongful Death Law." *Vanderbilt Law Review* 37 (March): 273–99.

Smeeding, Timothy M., ed. 1987. *Should Medical Care Be Rationed by Age?* Totowa, N.J.: Rowman and Littlefield.

Smith, Alwyn. 1987. "Qualms about QALYs." *Lancet,* May 16, pp. 1134–36.

Smith, George Teeling. 1985. *The Measurement of Health.* London: Office of Health Economics.

Smith, George Teeling, ed. 1984. *Measuring the Social Benefits of Medicine.* London: Office of Health Economics.

Somers, Anne R. 1982. "Long-Term Care for the Elderly and Disabled." *New England Journal of Medicine* 307 (July 22): 221–26.

Sowell, Thomas. 1984. "The Poor as Hostages: How to Justify Big Spending." *Seattle Times,* December 19, p. A15.

Specter, Michael. 1988. "Oregon Legislators Face Up to the Hard Job of 'Playing God.'" *Washington Post National Weekly Edition,* February 15–21, p. 33.

Speiser, S. M. 1970. *Recovery for Wrongful Death: Economic Handbook.* Rochester, Minn.: Lawyers Cooperative.

———. 1975. *Recovery for Wrongful Death,* 2d ed. Rochester, Minn.: Lawyers Cooperative.

Spicker, S. F., J. M. Healey, and H. T. Engelhardt, eds. 1981. *The Law-Medicine Relation: A Philosophical Exploration.* Dordrecht: D. Reidel.

Starzl, Thomas E. 1985. "Will Live Organ Donations No Longer Be Justified?" *Hastings Center Report* 15 (April): 5.

Stein, J. 1985. "Industry's New Bottom Line on Health Care Costs: Is Less Better?" *Hastings Center Report* 15 (October): 14–18.

Steinbock, Bonnie. 1986. "The Logical Case for 'Wrongful Life.'" *Hastings Center Report* 16 (April): 15–20.

Sterba, James P., ed. 1985. *The Ethics of War and Nuclear Deterrence*. Belmont, Calif.: Wadsworth.

Stern, Joanne B. 1983. "Will the Tort of Bad Faith Breach of Contract Be Extended to Health Maintenance Organizations?" *Law, Medicine and Health Care* 11 (February): 12–18, 21.

Stoddart, Greg L., et al. 1986. "Tobacco Taxes and Health Care Costs: Do Canadian Smokers Pay Their Way?" *Journal of Health Economics* 5 (March): 63–80.

Stone, Alan A. 1985. "Law's Influence on Medicine and Medical Ethics." *New England Journal of Medicine* 312 (January 31): 309–12.

Strong, Carson. 1983. "The Tiniest Newborns." *Hastings Center Report* 13 (February): 14–19.

Stuart, F. P. 1984. "Need, Supply, and Legal Issues Related to Organ Transplantation in the U.S." *Transplantation Proceedings* 16 (February): 87–94.

Stuart, F. P., et al. 1981. "Brain Death Laws and Patterns of Consent to Remove Organs from Cadavers in the United States and 28 Other Countries." *Transplantation* 31 (April): 238–44.

Sugden, Robert. 1983. *Who Cares? An Economic and Ethical Analysis of Private Charity and the Welfare State*. London: Institute of Economic Affairs.

———. 1985a. "Rejoinder" to Culyer and Posnett (1985). *Economic Affairs* 5 (January–March): 42.

———. 1985b. "Why Be Consistent? A Critical Analysis of Consistency Requirements in Choice Theory." *Economica* 52 (May): 167–83.

Terleckyj, Nesto E., ed. 1976. *Household Production and Consumption*. New York: National Bureau of Economic Research.

Thaler, Richard. 1982. "Precommitment and the Value of a Life." In Jones-Lee, ed., pp. 171–83.

———. 1987. "The Psychology of Choice and the Assumptions of Economics." Working Paper RR-3, Center for Philosophy and Public Policy, University of Maryland, College Park.

Thaler, Richard, and Sherwin Rosen. 1976. "The Value of Saving a Life." In Terleckyj, ed., pp. 265–98.

Thompson, Mary E., and William F. Forbes. 1982. "Costs and 'Benefits' of Cigarette Smoking in Canada." *Canadian Medical Association Journal* 127 (November 1): 831–32.

———. 1985. "Reasons for the Disagreements on the Impact of Smoking on Medical Care Expenditures: A Proposal for a Uniform Approach." *Social Science in Medicine* 21 (July): 771–73.

———. 1986. "Smoking and Medical Care Expenditures—What We Know and What We Don't Know." *Social Science in Medicine* 23 (January): 93–94.

Thomson, Judith Jarvis. 1985. "Imposing Risks." In Gibson, ed., pp. 125–40.

Thurow, Lester C. 1984. "Learning to Say 'No.'" *New England Journal of Medicine* 311 (December 13): 1569–72.

Titmuss, Richard M. 1971. *The Gift Relationship: From Human Blood to Social Policy.* New York: Vintage Books.

Tooley, Michael. 1972. "Abortion and Infanticide." *Philosophy and Public Affairs* 2 (Fall): 37–65.

———. 1983. *Abortion and Infanticide.* Oxford: Clarendon Press.

Torrance, George W. 1986. "Measurement of Health State Utilities for Economic Appraisal: A Review." *Journal of Health Economics* 5 (March): 1–30.

Trianosky, Gregory W. 1986. "Supererogation, Wrongdoing, and Vice: On the Autonomy of the Ethics of Virtue." *Journal of Philosophy* 84 (January): 26–40.

Tullock, Gordon. 1985. Letter. *New York Review,* June 13, 1985, p. 64.

Tversky, Amos, and Daniel Kahneman. 1981. "The Framing of Decisions and the Psychology of Choice." *Science* 211 (January 30): 453–58.

———. 1982. "Judgment under Uncertainty: Heuristics and Biases." In Kahneman, Slovic, and Tversky, eds., pp. 3–20.

Usher, Dan. 1985. "The Value of Life for Decision Making in the Public Sector." In Paul, Miller, and Paul, eds., pp. 168–91.

Veatch, Robert M. 1980. "Voluntary Risks to Health: The Ethical Issues." *Journal of the American Medical Association* 243 (January 4): 50–55.

———. 1981. *A Theory of Medical Ethics.* New York: Basic Books.

———. 1985. "Ethical Dilemmas of For-Profit Enterprise in Health Care." In Gray, ed., pp. 125–52.

———. 1986. "DRGs and the Ethical Reallocation of Resources." *Hastings Center Report* 16 (June): 32–40.

———. 1987. Reply to Morreim (1987). *Hastings Center Report* 17 (April): 45–46.

———. 1988a. "Justice and the Economics of Terminal Illness." *Hastings Center Report* 18 (August): 34–40.

———. 1988b. Reply to letter. *Hastings Center Report* 18 (April–May): 43–44.

Veatch, Robert M., and Carol Mason. 1987. "Hippocratic vs. Judeo-Christian Medical Ethics: Principles in Conflict." *Journal of Religious Ethics* 15 (Spring): 86–105.

Viscusi, W. Kip. 1978. "Labor Market Valuations of Life and Limb: Empirical Evidence and Policy Implications." *Public Policy* 26 (Summer): 359–86.

———. 1983. *Risk by Choice: Regulating Health and Safety in the Workplace.* Cambridge, Mass.: Harvard University Press.

Warner, Kenneth E. 1985. "Cigarette Advertising and Media Coverage of Smoking and Health." *New England Journal of Medicine* 312 (February 7): 384–88.

———. 1986. "Smoking and Health Implications of a Change in the Federal Cigarette Excise Tax." *Journal of the American Medical Association* 255 (February 28): 1028–32.

———. 1987. "Health and Economic Implications of a Tobacco-Free Society." *Journal of the American Medical Association.* 258 (October 16): 2080–86.

Warner, Kenneth E., et al. 1986. "Promotion of Tobacco Products: Issues and Policy Options." *Journal of Health Politics, Policy and Law* 11 (Fall): 367–92.

Weiland, D., et al. 1984. "Information on 628 Living-Related Kidney Donors at a

Single Institution, with Long-Term Follow-up in 472 Cases." *Transplantation Proceedings* 16 (February): 5–7.

Weinrib, Ernest J. 1980. "The Case for a Duty to Rescue." *Yale Law Journal.* 90 (December): 247–93.

Weinstein, Milton C., Donald Shepard, and Joseph Pliskin. 1975. "Decision-Theoretic Approaches to Valuing a Year of Life." Boston: Center for Analysis of Health Practices, Harvard School of Public Health.

Weir, Robert F. 1984. *Selective Nontreatment of Handicapped Newborns.* New York: Oxford University Press.

———. 1985. "Selective Nontreatment—One Year Later: Reflections and a Response." *Social Science and Medicine* 20 (November): 1109–17.

———. 1987. "Imperiled Newborns: Three Moves to the Left of Center." *Medical Humanities Review* 1 (January): 39–47.

Werthmann, Barbara. 1984. *Medical Malpractice Law: How Medicine Is Changing the Law.* Lexington, Mass. D. C. Heath.

Westen, Peter. 1985. "The Concept of Equal Opportunity." *Ethics* 95 (July): 837–50.

White, Robert. 1975. "Case Studies in Bioethics: A Demand to Die." *Hastings Center Report* 5 (June): 9–10.

Wikler, Daniel. 1987. Comment on Battin (1987). In Smeeding, ed., pp. 95–98.

———. 1988. "Ought the Young Make Health Care Decisions for Their Aged Selves?" *Journal of Medicine and Philosophy* 13 (February): 57–72.

Williams, Alan. 1981. "Welfare Economics and Health Status Measurement." In Perlman and van der Gaag, eds. pp. 271–81.

———. 1984. "The Economic Role of 'Health Indicators.'" In Smith, ed., 63–67.

———. 1985a. "Economics of Coronary Artery Bypass Grafting." *British Medical Journal* 291 (August 3): 326–29.

———. 1985b. "The Value of QALYs." *Health and Social Service Journal,* July 18, pp. 3–5.

———. 1985c. "Medical Ethics: Health Service Efficiency and Clinical Freedom." *Nuffield/York Portfolios,* no. 2. York, U.K.: Centre for Health Economics, University of York.

———. 1986a. "Health Economics: The Cheerful Face of the Dismal Science?" Address to the Annual Meeting of the British Association for the Advancement of Science, September 1–5.

———. 1986b. Letter. *British Medical Journal* 293 (August 2): 337–38.

———. 1987. Letter in reply to Smith (1987). *Lancet,* June 13, p. 1372.

Winslow, Gerald R. 1984. "From Loyalty to Advocacy: A New Metaphor for Nursing." *Hastings Center Report* 14 (June): 32–40.

Winslow, Gerald R. 1986. "Rationing and Publicity." In Agich and Begley, eds., pp. 199–216.

Woodfield, Alan E. 1984. "Costs and 'Benefits' of Cigarette Smoking in Canada: Comment." *Canadian Medical Association Journal* 130 (January 15): 118–20.

Wrenn, Keith. 1985. "No Insurance, No Admission." *New England Journal of Medicine* 312 (February): 373–74.

Wright, Virginia Baxter. 1986. "Will Quitting Smoking Help Medicare Solve Its Financial Problems?" *Inquiry* 23 (Spring): 76–82.

Yaari, M. E., and M. Bar-Hillel. 1984. "On Dividing Justly." *Social Choice and Welfare.* 1 (May): 1–24.

Zeckhauser, Richard, and Donald Shepard. 1976. "Where Now for Saving Lives?" *Law and Contemporary Problems* 40 (Autumn): 5–45.

Zelizer, Viviana A. 1978. "Human Values and the Market: The Case of Life Insurance and Death in 19th-Century America." *American Journal of Sociology* 84 (November): 591–610.

———. 1979. *Morals and Markets: The Development of Life Insurance in the United States.* New York: Columbia University Press.

———. 1985. *Pricing the Priceless Child: The Changing Value of Children.* New York: Basic Books.

Zimmerman, Roger. 1981. "Coercive Wage Offers." *Philosophy and Public Affairs* 10 (Spring): 121–45.

Index

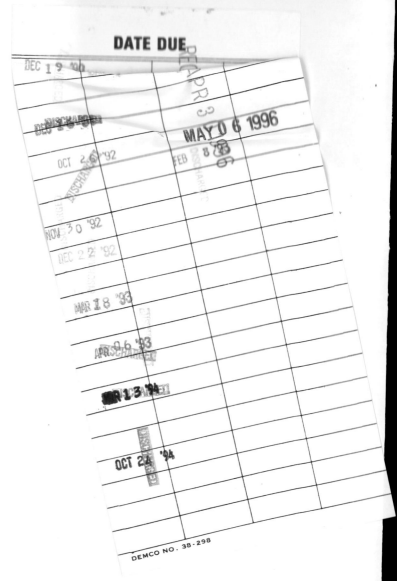